BOOMERCISE

Exercising as You Age

BOOMERCISE
Exercising as You Age

David Pargman, PhD

Emeritus professor, Florida State University

FITNESS INFORMATION TECHNOLOGY
A Division of the International Center
for Performance Excellence
West Virginia University
262 Coliseum, WVU-CPASS
PO Box 6116
Morgantown, WV 26506-6116

Library of Congress Card Catalog Number: 2011936287

ISBN: 978-1-935412-32-8

Cover photographs: (Front cover, clockwise from top right):
Moodboard_Images/iStockphoto.com; Monkey Business Images/
Dreamstime.com; Monkey Business Images/Dreamstime.com;
kzenon/www.123RF.com (Back cover, from left to right): Mark
Tilly/www.123RF.com; Monkey Business Images/Dreamstime.com;
Perkins8808/Dreamstime.com; Digoarpi/Dreamstime.com

Cover Design: Bellerophon Productions
Typesetter: Bellerophon Productions
Production Editor: Aaron Geiger
Copyeditor: Geoffry Fuller
Proofreader: Matt Brann
Indexer: Rachel Tibbs
Printed by: Data Reproductions Corp.

10 9 8 7 6 5 4 3 2 1

Fitness Information Technology
A Division of the International Center for Performance Excellence
West Virginia University
262 Coliseum, WVU-CPASS
PO Box 6116
Morgantown, WV 26506-6116
800.477.4348 (toll free)
304.293.6888 (phone)
304.293.6658 (fax)
Email: fitcustomerservice@mail.wvu.edu
Website: www.fitinfotech.com

CONTENTS

FOREWORD vii

PREFACE xi

CHAPTER SUMMARIES AND BOOK OUTLINE xv

CHAPTER 1: Why Exercise Is Important for Boomers 1

CHAPTER 2: Exercise, Wellness, Health, and Illness 37

CHAPTER 3: Eating Right and Feeling Good:
Nutritional Considerations 55

CHAPTER 4: Psychological Benefits of Exercise 79

CHAPTER 5: Avoiding Exercise Injury 103

CHAPTER 6: Exercise and Stress 123

CHAPTER 7: Staying with the Program: Not Quitting 147

CHAPTER 8: Setting Exercise Goals:
Establishing the Physical Activity Plan 167

CHAPTER 9: Choosing the Right Exercises for You 181

EPILOGUE: Final Food for Thought 209

GLOSSARY 211

REFERENCES 223

INDEX 227

ABOUT THE AUTHOR 231

FOREWORD

As a personal trainer, I find that Baby Boomers are one of the most rewarding populations to work with. They understand that exercise is not just about looking good in the mirror—it's about something that is much more meaningful and enjoyable. As we age, our priorities change, and Boomers are a prime example of a group of people who can find the richness and quality of life in some of life's simplicities that many younger people sometimes seem to overlook.

Early in my personal training career, I learned a valuable lesson from one of my clients. Each day I would work with this woman, and I soon realized that words like *progress*, *achievement*, and *accomplishment* were not defined by one specific meaning. My eyes were opened when my client shared with me that she was so excited that she could carry her bags of groceries up the stairs by herself without becoming fatigued. This accomplishment may seem insignificant to many people, but that moment taught me that it's the little things in life that make a big difference. My client found great joy in a personal achievement. She set a goal and accomplished it, and she rediscovered her independence. I felt greatly rewarded as I watched her accomplish a milestone in a grand journey of fitness and nutrition because I learned that while being able to carry bags of groceries up stairs without becoming tired isn't a milestone for everyone, for her it was a significant achievement and one that would have a direct and positive effect on her daily life.

As one of the trainers on NBC's "The Biggest Loser," I was able to witness similar milestones by the contestants who I worked with. Many were so overweight and out of shape when

they arrived at The Biggest Loser Ranch that they were unable to perform daily tasks that many people would take for
granted. But when I began to train the contestants and they altered their diet, I saw how excited they became not by being
able to perform rigorous exercises, but by being able to perform some of life's daily tasks that they previously were unable
to do.

Boomercise: Exercising as You Age can help you (and anyone else, for that matter) to gain more energy, improve your
health, and develop strength to do some of the "simple things"
in life that can be so rewarding. Whether your goals are to be
able to keep up with your grandchildren and carry them without pain and fatigue, or if your goals go into deeper levels of
fitness such as running a 5K race, the knowledge you will acquire from this book will help you to achieve your personal
milestones. *Boomercise* doesn't just tell you how to find those
joys that come with exercise and nutrition, it *shows* you. There
is truly something in here for everyone.

As with all people, Boomers have varying levels of fitness,
nutritional habits, and personal needs. My mother, Linda Schw-
erdt, is a woman who is functioning on a higher level of fitness.
She is 65 years old, and has her Red belt in karate. She can do
65 pushups. She takes walks regularly with my father, Gary.

But my mother didn't simply arrive at her current level of
fitness—she worked for it, step by step. *Boomercise* talks about
the necessity of setting goals, and of finding the right exercise
for you. My mother found martial arts, which also has a built-
in goal-setting system of belts, routines, physical achievements,
and cultural education. In order to get from the beginning
white belt to the coveted black belt, each student must go
through the ranking system. My mother also set additional
goals for herself—for instance, she wants to be able to do 100
pushups before she tries out for her black belt.

Boomercise also pays attention to a lot of the areas of exercise and fitness that we take for granted, such as the psychology of exercise. Author David Pargman takes careful note of

the importance of social psychology, or, simply put, the need for the mind to engage with others. My mother functions in a social setting. She actively and routinely engages with other people, even when going on those walks with my dad. When I work with my clients, either one-on-one or in a group setting, there is a lot of interactivity and accountability. The human mind is often overlooked when it comes to evaluating exercise and fitness, and is forgotten about in many books. I teach others that being healthy on the inside (mentally and psychologically) is one of the most important steps to feeling good on the outside (physically). As we age, our minds age right along with our bodies, so it's vital that we keep our minds healthy along with our bodies. How we view ourselves can make all of the difference in the world.

I suspect that some Boomers will be hesitant to read *Boomercise* because they'll dismiss themselves as being too old, frail, or feeble to get any results. During the aging process, it seems more difficult to rebound from the rigors of exercise that we once took for granted as young adults. But is it too late to start exercising? The answer is an emphatic "no!" From my experiences as a personal trainer and athlete, I've found that one of the immediate benefits from starting an exercise regimen is that you'll notice an increase in energy. And with that energy, you will be able to do more exercise, and more often. People need to realize that they need to move their bodies, and often. Although my mother's health is inspiring, many of her peers and friends are experiencing health issues—problems that could have been prevented or assisted simply by exercising and eating right. The combination of positive effects should be enough to motivate anyone to get up and move!

So take careful note of what *Boomercise* has to offer within these pages. Use your Boomer brain and lust for life to absorb the many aspects of exercise and fitness that *Boomercise* details: psychology, nutrition, planning, and even how different parts of the body functions on an individual level.

May I offer one last piece of advice? I'd like you to abandon any fear of failure that you may have. Get out there and enjoy your life and the lives of those you love.

Kim Lyons earned a reputation as a "no excuse" trainer on the NBC hit show "The Biggest Loser." She is a National Academy of Sports Medicine certified personal trainer with certifications in corrective exercise and sports performance who has been working with clients of all ages for more than a decade. She has also won several titles while competing in fitness competitions. Lyons is the author of *Your Body, Your Life*, which takes an uncomplicated approach to fitness and weight loss and is available through her website (www.kimlyons.com). She has appeared on television and in print, in such places as The Today Show, Larry King Live, Dr. Phil, *People Magazine*, *TV Guide*, *Women's World*, *US Weekly*, and many others.

PREFACE

We are designed to move, and move we must. Regardless of how we come to be endowed with some extraordinary motor abilities, the fact remains that we stand upright, rotate our arms, grasp objects, flex our knees, bend at the waist, and proceed forward, backwards, and sideways. We are privileged to move in these ways, but to sustain such abilities we must keep our muscles strong, our nervous system healthy, and our skeletal framework flexible and sound. To these ends, exercise is downright essential.

A great deal about the positive effects of exercise upon psychological health and general well-being are known and very honestly, quite impressive. We know, for instance, that regular physical activity is associated with reduced symptoms of anxiety and depression and that when done to certain degrees of intensity and performed in short periods of time, lowers stress levels. Frail, disabled, and challenged persons also improve in overall function through physical activity. AIDS victims, although not necessarily increasing their lifespan as a result of exercise, report an improved quality of life. Exercise makes them feel better and has a positive influence upon their outlook.

Here's the thing: You must add exercise to your litany of daily commitments. Exercise is a requirement, an essential part of your life. Its absence from your everyday "to do" lists ultimately deprives you of an optimally healthy existence. You can live without it, but life is infinitely improved with it. The situation is as straight forward and simple as that. And that's precisely what this book is all about.

Mind you, no one is asking you to run marathons or weight lift with 300 pounds. No one is suggesting that you cycle up steep mountains or kayak down treacherous cascades. What is being emphatically recommended in this book is regular participation in some sort of structured program of physical activity. My purpose in offering this small volume is to convince men and women who are a part of the Boomer generation or older that regular exercise is as essential to their well-being as proper nutrition, dental hygiene, a good night's rest, personal grooming, and avoidance of tobacco.

When I decided to put this book together I struggled with the trepidation that my cajoling would result in accusations of ranting zealotry. I hope that this is not the case. Of course I remain absolutely convinced of the criticality of exercise in all of our lives and have made an effort to back up my exhortations, admonitions, caveats, and claims with factual information stemming mostly from fairly recent scientific research. And I realize that my enthusiasm for delivering this message can on occasion be unbridled. But I believe that my argument needs to be heard, particularly by those in the Boomer generation—those men and women born a little after World War II. These adults still retain vitality and a capacity for physical activity, but in many cases they interpret my encouragement and similar advice from others as unrealistic and Herculean in nature. This is certainly not the case. I am entirely confident that my intended readership is not completely naïve about the physical and psychological benefits of exercise. However, for one reason or another, they have been unable or unwilling to take the plunge. Among the Boomer population there are certainly literate individuals who not only consume newspaper and magazine articles that speak to the need to be physically active, but also listen to and view countless television ads, programs, and messages that encourage them to get off their rear ends. In this book I try to get the Boomer-reader off the mark, to explain what exercise is and how it can assume various forms, how it can provide enormous benefits and how it can be the cherry on the ice cream sundae that life should be. In presenting my case,

I attempt to clarify misconceptions and defend worthwhile practices, while providing support that stems from my own experiences, my years of education and study, as well as from experts in the field. I provide guidelines intended to steer readers along the correct path. I offer general principles that should enable you to make *safe* and *sensible* (two words that I belabor throughout the book) decisions about the type, intensity, and frequency of physical activity that is best for you.

So much for what this book intends to accomplish. Now a brief word about what it is not. This is not a book that details specific movements illustrated by photographs of lean and muscular men and women. It does not offer stick figures, photographs, or diagrams of how to do a sit-up or biceps curl with weights. Such volumes are not without value, and they are legion in your local bookstore. But this is not what I'm offering. I'm presenting a case for exercise. I'm saying that people of approximately 60 years of age who no longer exercise regularly or who haven't been in a program for a long time need to get started again. *Now!*

With this in mind, I explain why you should start and show you how to get started. And for those of you who are already involved with regular exercise, the book provides an additional service: helping you discover whether what you are doing is prudent and safe. To this end I describe common pitfalls that tend to discourage regular participation or encourage quitting. I talk about your body's physiological functions, its various organs and systems, and the ways in which they are affected by physical activity. I discuss motivation, exercise as stress relief, protection from exercise-related injury, and the value of realistic and attainable exercise goals.

I hope I'm right about the importance and usefulness of this book. I wish you the very best and most enjoyable exercise experience possible.

CHAPTER SUMMARIES AND BOOK OUTLINE

Chapter 1: WHY EXERCISE IS IMPORTANT FOR BOOMERS

This chapter introduces you to the necessity of participating in regular exercise. The author makes the case for the positive influence of exercise upon mental and physical health and sets the stage for the book's basic thematic emphasis.

CONTENT SUMMARY:

- Exercise improves mental and physical health in older individuals more than in any other age group.
- Exercise reduces plaque in arteries and veins.
- Exercise exerts a positive influence on cognitive processes and can help manage anxiety and depression.
- Decline in certain mental abilities is slower among exercisers.
- Exercise helps manage body weight.
- Exercisers with high fitness levels have relatively stronger immune systems.
- Because many forms of exercise strengthen muscles that help maintain balance, exercise has long-term fall-prevention potential.

Chapter 2: EXERCISE, WELLNESS, HEALTH, AND ILLNESS

This chapter distinguishes among wellness, health, and illness, and establishes links between exercise and illness prevention,

and exercise and wellness. The author explains how many illnesses prevalent among elderly persons may be curtailed
through exercise.

CONTENT SUMMARY:

- Health and wellness are not the same. You can be well but
  not healthy, or you can be very healthy, but not well.
- Exercise has the capability to strengthen the immune system and keep natural protective mechanisms working on
  your behalf.
- Exercise can arrest encroaching osteoporosis.
- Obesity is a serious menace to your health and wellness.
  Diet is crucial, but exercise may contribute to the reduction of obesity.
- Exercise done wisely can help arthritic joints maintain
  looseness and lubrication.

Chapter 3: EATING RIGHT AND FEELING GOOD: NUTRITIONAL CONSIDERATIONS

The chapter begins with a discussion of body image—what we
believe we see when we look into the mirror—and details the
extent to which it influences our behavior and the way in which
we interact with others. The chapter then discusses how body
fat is stored and burned, and the various physical and psychological liabilities associated with being overweight. The chapter then addresses and debunks numerous persistent myths
pertaining to nutrition and diet, focusing specifically on the nutritional requirements of older persons. Finally, the chapter addresses the advisability of so-called *nutritional supplements*.

CONTENT SUMMARY:

- *Body image* is the view we hold of our physical selves and
  is fundamental to our wellness, health, and happiness.
- What foodstuffs, and in what specific amounts, does your

body require for good health and wellness? Using information and advice in this chapter, you will be able to answer these questions. You have little control over your body height or natural eye color, but you can regulate what you eat.

- Your exercise program should be carefully coordinated with a sensible diet.

Chapter 4: PSYCHOLOGICAL BENEFITS OF EXERCISE

As we age, some of our intellectual capacities lose sharpness. This chapter provides evidence that participation in regular, appropriately prescribed physical activity may slow such change. Thinking and remembering may be improved as a consequence of exercise participation.

CONTENT SUMMARY:

- Both mind and brain function tend to decrease somewhat as we age.
- Exercise improves brain and mind activity and inhibits their deterioration.
- A personality profile may help determine what kind of exercise is best for you.
- For many physiological reasons, exercise improves your mood.

Chapter 5: AVOIDING EXERCISE INJURY

Exercise programs should be custom made, accommodating individual participants and their particular needs and interests. The longer we live, the more we accumulate a variety of limitations and disabilities—minor though they may be—as a result of traumas, career, or work-related mishaps or misuse of body parts. This chapter provides advice enabling you to make prudent decisions about the kind of exercise that is least likely to make things worse and most likely to be wholesome and beneficial.

CONTENT SUMMARY:

- During or as a consequence of rigorous exercise, injury may occur. The best we can do is make informed decisions in order to reduce the likelihood of injury.

- Too much of a good thing can be problematical and too much exercise can be injurious. Exercisers need to schedule their activities effectively and exercise with appropriate intensity.

- All individual Boomers are unique, no matter how similar their age. You, therefore, require tailor-made exercise prescriptions; learn what types of activities are compatible with special needs and goals.

- Stretching is an essential physical activity for people over 60.

Chapter 6: EXERCISE AND STRESS

This chapter clarifies the relationship between exercise and the stress response. It begins with a discussion of stress—its causes and consequences—and describes the ways stress can be positive as well as negative. The chapter explains how and why exercise is a crucial component of any stress-control regimen.

CONTENT SUMMARY:

- You can learn how to control your body's reaction to events that provoke stress reactions. You can manage your stress responses so that they benefit you. You can learn to harness the potential power and positive force of stress. Exercise is a strategy for accomplishing this.

- When done improperly or excessively, exercise may heighten your stress response and thus be detrimental.

Chapter 7: STAYING WITH THE PROGRAM: NOT QUITTING

Structure your exercise environment appropriately to increase the likelihood of sticking with your program. Be realistic when determining the best time of day for exercise and consider all the variables when creating your exercise regimen. Are you a morning person? When do you feel strongest? What time of day are you most productive? How far must you travel to exercise? Will you be able to find a partner every time? Will the traffic be a formidable obstacle? Is the selected route for your walk workout safe? Can you handle the terrain? What will a spate of inclement weather do if gardening is your preferred physical activity? This chapter helps you think through all the details you need to consider.

CONTENT SUMMARY:

- In order to maintain a high level of motivation for exercise participation, it is important to fully understand your reason for entering the program in the first place.

- Dropping out is a major problem for exercisers. Certain strategies can reduce the likelihood of quitting.

- It is critical that you know how long to exercise and when to stop, but in order to derive optimal benefit you must stick to it. Exercise should be done regularly.

Chapter 8: SETTING EXERCISE GOALS: ESTABLISHING THE PHYSICAL ACTIVITY PLAN

In this chapter you are encouraged to determine exactly what you wish to accomplish during any of your exercise bouts. How long will you participate? How many successive repetitions will you accomplish? What distance will you cover? These determinations are known as exercise goals and should be established on a personal basis. What may be an appropriate goal for one exerciser may not be indicated for another.

CONTENT SUMMARY:

- Goal-setting assists exercisers in sustaining high levels of motivation and in participating in safe and appropriate activities.

- Goals should be realistic and attainable.

- Goals should also be evaluated regularly and reset when appropriate.
- Good goal-setting will result in high levels of motivation for exercise and thus, regularity of participation.

Chapter 9: CHOOSING THE RIGHT EXERCISES FOR YOU

This chapter provides guidelines for selecting physical activities that are best for individual exercisers. Personal prescriptions are not given and you are encouraged to utilize the principles and guidelines to establish your own regimen of exercise. What is good for the goose is not necessarily good for the gander, and you are encouraged to arrange for a program of physical activity that suits you and satisfies your individual needs and interests.

CONTENT SUMMARY:

- The appropriate form of exercise depends upon your current fitness needs and objectives.
- For overall fitness your program should be comprehensive and address strength, endurance, agility, flexibility, and aerobic capacity.
- The importance of stretching should be acknowledged when constructing the individual exercise program. Stretching should be done strategically and knowledgeably.
- Exercise machines can be safe and helpful.
- Dress appropriately for out of doors exercise.
- Running is not a good activity for everyone. Jogging or walking is preferable for most exercisers as they age.

Chapter I

WHY EXERCISE IS IMPORTANT FOR Boomers

Harry is 75 years old and has never exercised. He never felt that cavorting in shorts or pushing weights in a gym was his cup of tea. He worked hard for many years as an accountant, putting in long hours in his office in order to provide for his wife and children. He was never interested in physical labor for fun. With tongue in cheek he maintains he has lived successfully, healthfully, and happily for 75 years without exercise, and at this age, he sees no reason to begin.

Harry is dead wrong. Despite not exercising regularly in the past, Harry would reap beneficial and impressive results at the age of 75 if he were to begin an exercise program immediately. Trite as it may seem, when it comes to exercise, it is never too late to get started. If you've never exercised regularly but get off the mark now, within weeks you'll notice significant and desirable changes. I say this not only as a person with more than 70 years of living under my belt and with decades of personal exercise experience to my credit but because a solid scientific basis exists for this claim. A stream of testimonials and support from a variety of sources surfaces daily and em-

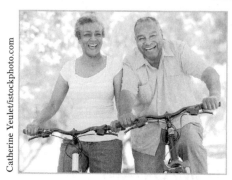

Catherine Yeulet/istockphoto.com

In spite of what you may think, it is never too late to get started exercising. Within weeks you'll be able to notice significant changes.

phatically informs us that the evidence is especially impressive for older individuals. And older adults increasingly cope with health challenges that don't surface as frequently in pre-Boomer years. In a recent interview synopsized in the *New York Times Magazine*,[1] Dr. Regina Benjamin, the United States Surgeon General, refers to exercise as medicine. She says, "It's better than most pills."

If you were born between the years 1946 and 1964 you're a Boomer. People satisfying this U.S. Census imposed criterion are expected to live another 18 to 20 years—another 20 more years of excitement, fulfillment, pleasure, well being, and good health. That is, if you nourish and protect your health and strive to strengthen it further. Exercise can be invaluable in this regard. If you can get off the easy chair and tap into this potential fountain of youth you can live longer and reduce the chances of disability, stroke, mental deterioration, and type 2 diabetes. Here's the bottom line: If you don't move regularly and vigorously, if you cling to the couch and wallow in the sedentary life, you are risking a future of very poor health.

In a March 2008 article in the *New York Times* titled "The Cure for Exhaustion? More Exercise," the journalist Tara Parker-Pope talks about findings reported by University of Georgia researchers who learned that 20 minutes of moderate intensity aerobic exercise, three times a week for six weeks, had a very positive effect on reported energy levels in people suffering from feelings of fatigue. This may be surprising because one would be inclined to assume that exercise contributes to fatigue rather than alleviating it. This is not the case, and regular physical activity has recently been identified by William Thies, chief medical and scientific officer of the Alzheimer's Association, as one of a number of lifestyle characteristics that could reduce the risk of brain decline.[2] In fact, the article goes on to report that in both men and women 65 years and older, those who participated in moderate to heavy levels of physical activity had a whopping 40% lower risk for any type of dementia. In other words, you can slow down your brain's aging by incorporating regular exercise into your lifestyle. Even the most ardent skeptics should be impressed by such findings.

In this chapter and throughout the book, I'll occasionally share some of this evidence and argue that you are seriously short-changing yourself without regular exercise in your life. Regardless of how content you are without regular physical activity, exercise will elevate your quality of life. I'll even go as far as to say that for most of us, life cannot be fully satisfying without it. Exercise is preventive medicine and should be a part of your life.

A carefully planned and executed physical activity program can open doors to friendships and social contacts you have not previously explored. Exercise can significantly help regulate body weight, prevent or control diabetes, and strengthen your immune system to improve your ability to ward off infection and illness. In study after study, report after report, and article after article, older persons who have begun to exercise report meaningful changes in overall contentment, as well as a boost to energy levels. Problematic aging often involves physical inactivity, so choosing to exercise is the most effective decision you can make about your health. If a key to anti-aging exists, it is exercise.

As we age we lose muscle mass, muscle strength, muscle and tendon flexibility, and bone tissue. But the sharpness of this decline may be countered or delayed by exercise, thus preventing loss of mobility and reduced functional independence. If you are already physically active, consider cranking up your effort. By increasing the duration or speed of your exercise, you may even benefit more.

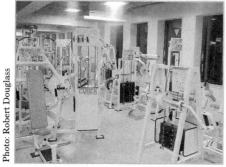

Photo: Robert Douglass

Regular physical activity reduces the risk of premature mortality in general, and of coronary heart disease, hypertension, colon cancer, and diabetes mellitus in particular.

—Surgeon General Regina M. Benjamin

Rigorous Whole-Body Physical Activity

Your body is capable of moving in many different and fascinating ways. But the speed, strength, and efficiency with which it alters its position in space depend upon your individual physical characteristics and the demands of a particular situation. You are by nature taller, heavier, more muscular than some people and thinner, shorter, and less muscular than others. All of us have our own special movement patterns just as we have our personal voice pitches and hair color.

If we are of sound body, we can move—in specific situations we do so in certain ways. When we dance with a partner, we use our arms and hands quite differently than when we are lining up a golf putt. Our muscular efforts are quite different when we swim than when we wield a rake. Not only do we move because the design of our body permits and encourages us to do so, but our bodies need physical activity and benefit from it in both the long and short term. Listen once more to the words of Regina M. Benjamin, Surgeon General of the United States. In her 1996 report titled "Physical Activity and Health," she states that "regular physical activity reduces the risk of premature mortality in general, and of coronary heart disease, hypertension, colon cancer, and diabetes mellitus in particular." What more of a message and inspiration could you possibly require?

As Time Goes By

As we age we tend to become less fit unless an effort is made to prevent this from occurring. And after age 45 the down-slide accelerates. According to Drs. Marco Pahor of the University of Florida and Jeff Williamson of Winston-Salem State University, cardiorespiratory fitness, in particular, declines more rapidly than other elements after the age of 45. In addition, decreased heart and lung function correlates strongly with the presence of diseases that limit our daily activity. According to Pahor and Williamson, in older adults physical inactivity "is perhaps the root cause of many unnecessary and premature admissions to long-term care." And Miriam E. Nelson, Director of the John Hancock Center for Physical Activity and Nutrition at Tufts University in Boston, offers this observation in the Fall, 2010 issue of *The Journal of Active Aging*: "With every increasing decade of age, people become less and less active." A reasonable, even undeniable offshoot of this observation is that exercise becomes more necessary as the decades pass.

In a *New York Times Personal Health* section 3, columnist Jane E. Brody wrote, "Every hour of the day, 330 Americans turn 60; by 2030 one in five Americans will be older than 65; the number of people over 100 doubles every decade."

Though you may already be 60 or older, now's the time to establish your very own program. In fact, if you are of this vintage, a sensible exercise routine, custom-made to your special needs and interests, is not only critical to your physical well-being but also to your psychological well-being. And here's something else that may surprise you: *exercise has been shown to improve mental and physical health in older individuals more than in any other age group.* All age groups benefit appreciably from exercise, but older persons do so more positively and dramatically. Why? Perhaps their baseline or beginning fitness is so much lower than that of other age groups that when they eventually become active, the results are more striking.

Boomer Fitness: A Personal Matter

As a starting point, let's agree upon the meaning of the term *exercise* because we'll be talking about this behavior incessantly from here on in. I recommend that you *think of exercise as rigorous physical activity done to improve some aspect of physical fitness*. And as far as the term *fitness* is concerned, although we'll cover this topic in considerable detail in Chapter 2, for now think of it as simply referring to *your ability to do what your daily agenda requires*. Examples of daily needs are cleaning out the garage, shoveling snow from the driveway, mowing the lawn, lifting grandchildren, stretching to retrieve a can of soup from the pantry shelf, and carrying a piece of fairly heavy luggage at the airport. The term *fitness* refers to your readiness to do such things and meet these kinds of challenges with comfort and dispatch. When you have sufficient strength, agility, power, endurance, and flexibility to do these things—that is, the jobs that are required of you on a regular basis—then you are fit. Fitness is idiosyncratic, highly personal. Your fitness needs are unique to you. Not all of the activities in which you choose to engage cover all dimensions of fitness. Reaching for a can of soup located on a high pantry shelf may not require a great deal of agility, but it taps into flexibility and muscular endurance. And lifting a fallen toddler would probably not place significant demands upon agility, but it places a premium on strength and power. When we use the word *exercise*, the implication is that at least one or more of the core elements of fitness are being addressed. We'll return to these two concepts in the next chapter.

Biological Organization: A Systems Approach

By now you should have gotten my fundamental point: exercise is more than merely important. It's absolutely vital. But how exactly how does this work? What are the mechanisms by which exercise accomplishes its magic? For this to be thoroughly understood, it is necessary to review the way the body is put together and consider the functions of each of its major biological systems. You can appreciate the positive impact of regular physical activity by understanding how your body's notable organs and systems function.

Although eight systems serve us (circulatory, respiratory, skeletal, muscular, nervous, endocrine, digestive, excretory), I'll deal only with the five systems that are most directly affected by exercise. No one is asking you to study intricate anatomical details, nor will any be provided. No exam will be administered and no final grades given. But you need to appreciate your body's marvelous arrangement of muscles and bones, glands and organs, and the incredible way they work together to ensure your health and well-being. In one way or another, these functions are the essence of our existence and contribute to our uniqueness as human beings. Only when we are able to understand basic biological operations can we value and admire how they are influenced by physical activity. If you are already in touch with what follows, don't fret. A light and brief review of what you may have studied years ago in junior or senior high school will stand you in good stead. To ease your reading, I've italicized words that require your special attention.

Now let's consider specific systems. I'll keep the review short and simple. But remember that these mechanisms operate in all of us who are physiologically sound, whether we are under or over 60 years of age. We begin with the circulatory system.

BLOOD VESSELS, BLOOD FLOW, PLAQUE, AND EXERCISE

The elixir of life, blood brings vital goodies including the essential gas, oxygen, to your needy body tissues. It is pumped and distributed by a perpetually beating (about 100,000 times a day), fist-size muscle located in the center of your chest, the heart. The tubes through which blood flows vary in size but must remain flexible, clear, and open. However, at age 60 and beyond these desired tubular characteristics are likely to be somewhat compromised, impeding blood flow to some degree.

Your Boomer arteries and veins lose some of their elasticity as they age, and their interior walls become lined with a fatty material known as *plaque*, which is related to the amount of cholesterol present in your blood over many years. These changes tend to elevate blood pressure—a common consequence of aging—and account for more beats per minute in the Boomer heart than in young adults. Twenty- or thirty-year-olds usually have more healthy arteries and veins than older persons, and therefore, the supply of blood necessary for optimal functioning of their body cells is delivered more easily and effectively.

Certain body organs can work reasonably well despite diminished blood circulation, but others, such as the brain, suffer dire consequences when flow is reduced even briefly. Brain cells die within minutes when deprived of oxygen. Aging takes a natural toll on the circulatory system, but as you'll see later in the chapter, exercise can keep your blood vessels clear and healthy. Here's something to remember and perhaps pass on to near and dear ones of younger years: Circulatory slow-down doesn't begin in Boomerhood. Inactivity in the 20s and 30s sets the stage for problematic blood flow in later years. Teenagers, 20- and 30-year-olds are not guaranteed perfectly functioning cardiac and circulatory systems by virtue of their age. They, too, should attend to the necessity of being physically active. But aging does bring with it a greater probability of circulatory impairment and a greater imperative to do something about it.

Not only are vital materials dispersed to your body's tissues, but waste products of your cellular activities are collected by the blood during its journey. This detritus is then transported by the blood to various organs for excretion. Blood thus has both a delivery function, akin to that of your mail carrier, and a garbage collection function like that provided by your waste disposal service. You need both to maintain a household that is tidy and in constant communication with others who have important information to exchange and provide. When you are involved in exercise, all these important operations accelerate. Your muscles produce increased amounts of waste and require additional supplies of fuel and oxygen. Therefore, you breathe more rapidly and deeply and your heart beats faster.

A sound circulatory system is a closed system. This means

that blood moves in a predetermined direction, taking oxygen and other nourishment to the body's cells and collecting waste materials. Although its contents change, the same blood moves all around your body. Blood consists mostly of water and is manufactured by special body organs. Think of your automobile's air-conditioning mechanism, which is also a closed system. When it's working properly, no coolant is lost and cooled air keeps circulating. When the system breaks down, air or coolant leaks and you're in trouble.

A few important facts: When you exercise, your heart thumps faster than when you are at rest. At rest its rate is somewhere around 60–80 beats per minute, depending upon your level of fitness and your sex. Women tend to have more rapid *pulses* than men. Your pulse is the sound of blood slamming against the wall of an artery. The more rapid the heart rate, the faster your pulse. During rigorous exercise, such as shoveling snow or raking leaves, your pulse can exceed 100 beats per minute. Naturally, during sleep your resting heart rate slows. After participating in exercise, especially aerobic exercise, on a regular basis for an extended period of time—perhaps two or three months—your heart becomes efficient and ejects a greater amount of blood at each heartbeat. Thus, it is able to beat fewer times each minute. The heart rate or pulse of a trained person tends therefore to be lower than that of an untrained or poorly fit individual.

What's your pulse? A convenient location for determining your heart rate is on the wrist. Place your index and middle fingers of the right hand on your left wrist below the base of the left thumb. When you sense rhythmical beats in your fingers check your watch or available timepiece and count your pulse for 60 seconds, or multiply a 15-second count by four. Note of the number of beats in the allocated time so you can use this number in the future to see if it decreases after two months of your exercise program. You can also see if your heart rate differs from your resting pulse immediately after exercising. Your *aerobic capacity* is the ability of your cardiovascular system to deliver oxygen to the body's cells during exercise. Fit persons therefore have greater aerobic capacities. In order to improve your aerobic capacity, it's necessary to engage regularly in some sort of aerobic training, training that taxes the cardiorespiratory mechanisms for about 20 to 30 minutes.

Target heart rate is a term used to refer to your appropriate training zone or the rate at which your heart should beat. Here's how you calculate it: subtract your chronological age from 220 (supposedly the highest heart rate typically achieved by humans) and then determine somewhere between 60 and 80% of this figure, depending upon how hard you wish to work and what you believe your fitness level happens to be. Here are step-by-step directions to determining the target heart rate for a 70-year-old person.

1. Subtract your age (70) from an arbitrary heart rate of 220. The result is 150.

2. Now multiply 150 by .60, .70, or .80; each of which represents the percent of effort you intend to put forth during exercise. If you multiplied by .60, you intend to put forth 60% effort during exercise and your target heart rate would be 90 beats per minute. The target heart rate at 80% effort would be 120.

3. The number you have derived after the multiplication represents the heart rate (number of beats per minute) that you should sustain for about 20 to 30 minutes of aerobic exercise. You should shoot for three aerobic workouts per week in the beginning.

If you selected the low end of the zone, 60% your pulse doing aerobic exercise would have been 90 (heart rate of 90 beats per minute). If you've not done aerobic exercise for a long time or consider yourself to be of relatively low fitness, use 50% in your calculation. After a number of training sessions you should know how it feels to exercise at your target heart rate. As you exercise pay attention to your breathing rate and your general impressions about the effort required to keep you in your zone for about 20 to 30 minutes. This is known as your *perceived exertion*. Or you can actually take your pulse during the training bout. Do this by counting the heart beats in a 15-second period and then multiply this number by four (4) to arrive at the number of beats per minute. You'll notice that when you eventually achieve a high level of aerobic fitness during exercise your heart rate will not elevate to the extent it did prior to your getting in shape. In addition, your pulse will return to its resting level sooner after exercise.

Another term used to describe the intensity of your exercise effort is *METs* or *metabolic equivalents*. You might come across this term in future readings or hear about it in the gym. The term is also used when your cardiologist administers a stress test on the treadmill. At three METs your effort is equivalent to three times your resting metabolic rate. Three to six METs is considered moderate exercise. Cycling more than 10 miles-per-hour would score more than six METs. Singles in tennis would also yield an excess of six METs depending upon your age and the length of time you played.

As mentioned previously, during aging the arteries and veins lose elasticity. Their interior walls also become lined with a fatty material known as plaque, which is related to the amount of cholesterol present in your blood over many years. Regular exercisers tend to have comparatively lower amounts of plaque in their arteries and veins.

Exercise also increases the amount of an important substance found in your blood. HDL, or high density lipoprotein, "washes away" plaque and thus prevents it from adhering to the walls of arteries and veins. Think of a garden hose whose insides are coated with sticky sludge that reduces water flow. The same is true with arteries and veins and blood flow. Regular exercisers tend to have less blood vessel sludge. When your hoses are clogged, less nutrients and oxygen are transported to brain cells. The sludge thickens and compromises the effectiveness of your blood vessels as conduits for the flow of brain necessities. In other words, the brain isn't getting what it needs to function effectively.

The degree to which your blood vessels clog depends upon a number of things: your genes, your lifestyle, and your diet. Genetic make-up, over which you have absolutely no control, conceivably regulates the extent to which blood vessels change and deteriorate (children don't have varicose veins). However, you are very much in control of your lifestyle and diet. One prominent theory on aging has it that your body cells are programmed to wear out over time and the length of time varies from person to person. Participation in an intensive exercise program may actually slow aging by influencing certain aspects of DNA function in cells of the cardiovascular system.

DNA, or deoxyribonucleic acid, is located in the nuclei of all your body's cells and is the basis for your hereditary endowment—what you get from your parents. But many scientists believe that lifestyle factors interacting with your personality traits (tendencies to think and behave in certain ways) can counterbalance or at least influence this genetic programming. This suggests that you indeed have some control over the situation.

You can choose to exercise because among other benefits, exercise can "rotor-rooter" your blood vessels. Vessels that are relatively clear and elastic facilitate desirable blood pressure, the force exerted against the vessel wall by the blood in keeping with the heart beat. In turn, appropriate blood pressure is associated with desirable blood distribution to the brain. In the long run, this results in less deterioration in mental function.

As previously described, you can slow down your brain's aging by incorporating regular exercise into your lifestyle. The better your brain circulation, the better your mental processes. Active adults of all ages—men as well as women—have lower incidents of heart attacks and strokes. In her column in the *New York Times*, Jane Brody puts matters into a perspective with which I'm entirely comfortable. She writes, "Regular exercise is the only well-established fountain of youth, and it's free."[4]

When people claim they feel better as a result of maintaining a regular exercise program, one aspect of this perception is undoubtedly improved circulatory function.

THE RESPIRATORY SYSTEM

Humans continually use *oxygen* and produce the waste gas, *carbon dioxide*. During exercise, more oxygen is needed because the muscles and other organs and systems of the body require increased amounts of fuel to function. Greater concentrations of waste products such as carbon dioxide appear in the blood and activate special centers in the brain that responsively trigger increased lung (*pulmonary*) activity.

Oxygen is found in the air you breathe and brought into the lungs during the process of *respiration*. You breathe more deeply and rapidly during exercise than when at rest.

Air from the environment enters through the mouth and nose and passes down the *trachea*, a tube whose origin is in the rear of the mouth. Your trachea divides into two branches: each leading to one of two lungs located in the chest cavity. Little air sacs known as *alveoli*, which comprise the lungs, fill with air. Oxygen, in the tiny and very thin-walled blood vessels called *capillaries* surrounding the alveoli, makes it way to the heart and ultimately into the blood, which transports it to all the body cells. A reverse procedure accounts for the movement of waste gases produced by cellular activity (*metabolism*)—that is, through the blood, capillaries, alveoli, trachea, and so forth.

Exercise—such as walking, gardening, or playing golf—that permits you to breathe regularly at will, is known as *aerobic*. When you swim across the pool underwater after taking a huge gulp of air, you are performing an *anaerobic* (without air) activity. When you struggle to open the unyielding lid from a vacuum-sealed jar of spaghetti sauce, you do so without benefit from a steady inflow of environmental air and the valuable oxygen it contains. In such situations your skeletal muscles are fortified by oxygen they have stored previously or which is kept in various biological warehouses in the body.

The amount of oxygen in storage is limited, and after a while you simply run out. Your gas tank is depleted, your working body parts no longer have adequate fuel to continue and you are unable to, or have difficulty expelling waste gas. You're out of breath. You gasp and quit. But some people are able to bring in more environmental air than others. They are said to have higher *max VO$_2$* capacities. Max VO$_2$ is determined by heredity and indicates the volume of oxygen you are able to inspire and use within a specified period of time. But it may be increased though training. If you don't try to maintain your max VO$_2$ level (whatever it may be) it will decrease with aging (about 1% per year after age 40).

THE NERVOUS SYSTEM

Your nervous system regulates all bodily functions, including muscular action. It is vital in acquiring and performing sport and recreational skills. In learning to fly-cast, shoot an arrow at a target, pitch a horseshoe, or swing a golf club, the nervous system is not only activated, but plays a primary role. For that matter, most any kind of learning and performing involves the nervous system. Although aging tends to take the sharp edge off its capacities, regular participation in a properly prescribed and administered program of physical activity can significantly inhibit this decline and perhaps even improve nervous system function.

Think of the nervous system in terms of two separate portions: the *sensory portion* and the *motor portion*. The responsibility of the sensory portion is to gather stimuli (signals) from outside the body and deliver them to the spinal cord and brain, known collectively as the central nervous system. Environmental stimuli surround you. They enter your nervous system through a variety of sensory pathways, namely visual (eyes), auditory (ears), tactile (touch), and so on.

Sensory nerves are positioned throughout your body in all the vital organs. They bring messages to the spinal cord, which is enclosed in the spinal (or *vertebral*) column. They then travel up the cord and very quickly reach the brain, where they are scanned, sorted, and stored. Some are kept in storage forever and some are buried so deeply in memory that they are difficult to access. The brain deposits these messages in special centers (where they become memories). At appropriate times they provide specific instructions to all of your bodily organs whose activation and involvement is required to deal with the situation at hand. For instance, the brain may transmit a signal to the heart to beat faster or slower when rigorous physical activity is begun or stopped. Such instructions are known as *motor stimuli*. They travel down the cord, communicate with the organs and related body parts, and provoke them into actually doing something about the incoming sensory stimuli already processed. Think of these sensory messages as those coming in to the brain (sensations from events going on all around you), and motor messages as those going out from the brain to all organs and systems of your body.

Your nerve cells connect with each other in long chains, and thus form complex communication networks. One nerve cell communicates with another at a location known as a *synapse*. Message transmission occurs in two ways: by electrical and chemical means. One nerve cell deposits a chemical substance on specialized receiving parts of another. Electrical current is also transferred from cell to cell. All of this "cell talk" happens in a flash, real fast. When you are involved in the type of physical activity we speak of in this book, namely exercise, your body requires stimulation that not only prepares it for action, but also keeps it going throughout the entire experience. Specially learned body movements, increased breathing, heart rate, and sweating to cool the body are but a few examples of mechanisms and actions that are triggered by nervous system message.

You are also able to regulate many nervous commands at will. You can learn to slow down or speed up some of them, just as you are able to consciously regulate the rate at which you walk. You can learn to do this by introducing thoughts or recollections of exiting or quieting experiences, thereby altering the characteristics of the messages. Your muscles and lungs will respond accordingly. Fortunately, many functions of the nervous system are both automatic and protective. They just happen without your provocation or interference. Through training you may be able to influence the rate at which your heart beats, but the brain automatically controls its very beating. It's not necessary for you to instruct your heart to beat.

An additional function of the nervous system involves certain products manufactured in special brain centers. I'll further develop this notion when I discuss psychological benefits of exercise in Chapter 7. But suffice to say at this point, the amount of chemical products such as *serotonin, dopamine, beta-endorphins*, and *enkephalin*, found in your bloodstream and in other locations in your body, changes significantly during exercise. These biochemicals are of the feel-good type. The more you have of them, the more you are emotionally satisfied.

All of the systems we've so far discussed, as well as the ones we've not yet gotten to, are interrelated. Their relationships are quite complex. When one system is weakened, others are usually affected and somehow compromised. A deteriorating circulatory system, for instance, reduces the efficiency of blood distribution, which in turn negatively affects the functioning of the muscular system. Because blood flow is impeded, muscles have difficulty getting rid of chemical waste products. This makes the muscles tire easily, and vital muscle groups, such as those involved in breathing, find it difficult to keep up your breathing rate and volume. Or if your immune system is weakened or otherwise functioning poorly, certain skeletal system operations become impaired, which may reult in, say, rheumatoid arthritis. The five systems selected here for your consideration are the ones most directly involved with exercise, but if you have the time and interest, you might also read about the fascinating contributions to your health and well-being made by the *endocrine*, *digestive*, and *excretory systems*. This is not to suggest that the organs in these systems are not at all involved in exercise—they most certainly are—but their contributions are not as dramatic or critical as the ones included in this chapter. Now let's examine two more very pertinent biological systems and their relationship to exercise, two that I've already alluded to: the *skeletal* and *muscular* systems.

THE SKELETAL SYSTEM

The skeleton is a collection of more than 600 bones that serves as a supportive foundation for your body parts. The long bones, such as the arms and legs, act as levers during movement. While exercising, it is the skeletal system that changes its position in space. Some bones are flat, and some are round and long. Some, such as the ribs, are curved and form a cage in which the heart and lungs are located for their protection. Other bones, such as the ones located in the middle of the ear, are tiny. The size and shape of bones indicate what they are prepared to do for you.

Bones meet at *joints*. *Ligaments*, constructed of thick, fibrous material, connect bones to other bones. Some joints bend in only one direction (for example, the knee), while others, such as the hip, have a wide range of motion. The design of a joint permits various forms of movement. Lubricating fluid and shock-absorbing tissues in joints enable their smooth function. When this fluid is depleted or the special tissue damaged, your joint may become irritated. This is indicative of one form of *arthritis*, known as osteoarthritis. Understandably, Boomer joints and bones have more mileage on them than those of 20-, 30-, or 40-year-olds. Keeping the skeletal system dense and the connective tissues (ligaments and tendons) strong and flexible through exercise goes a long way toward preventing or alleviating arthritis.

Limbs are attached to the skeleton at two wide and flat boney girdles, the *pectoral* and the *pelvic*. Your arms are attached to the pectoral girdle and legs to the pelvic girdle. This is true for all of us, but other characteristics of the skeletal system, such as length and width of bones, are determined by hereditary factors and vary from person to person. As you develop from early childhood to young adulthood, you undoubtedly become familiar with the mechanics of your basic movements. You learn about how your skeleton responds as your brain commands it to move. Much of what transpires during exercise is fundamentally related to how your bones function. When miscalculations are made about how to manage your skeletal system during rigorous physical activity, the result may be injury (which will be discussed in greater detail in Chapter 8). This is particularly true in activities that tend to place unusual stress upon the bones such as contact sports. Young bones are supple and pliable. They don't break as easily as the more brittle skeletal parts characteristic of elderly individuals. Toddlers are first becoming familiar with their skeletal responses as they move in space. But as an adult, you should be in touch with the capacities of your bone-levers as they lift objects and move your body during work and exercise.

THE MUSCULAR SYSTEM

More than 400 muscles are involved in your body's movement
in space. Those with primary responsibilities during exercise
are known as *skeletal muscles*. Most of these are attached to
tendons, which are tough, fibrous, connective tissues that function like rubber bands and attach muscle to bone. When skeletal muscles *contract* (this term usually, but not always, means
shorten) the tendons pull on the attached bone, which then
moves. Your arms' *biceps* muscles are good examples of this
action. They are connected to both upper arm and forearm.
When your biceps contract, the forearm is drawn toward the
upper arm. Skeletal muscles enable movement to occur, movement of limbs and movement of your body in space.

As is the case with bones, skeletal muscles are of various
shapes and sizes, which correspond to the type of function they
perform. Some are flat and wide; others are full in their middle
portions and tapered at both ends. Most skeletal muscles are
said to be *voluntary* because they respond to voluntary nervous stimuli in order to contract. In other words, you decide to
swing the golf club or pull on the rowboat's oars and then actually perform accordingly. This is not true of other kinds of
muscles that function on an automatic or *reflexive* basis. You
are unable to voluntarily control your eye blink at all times.
When someone moves a finger in your eye's direction the lid
protectively and automatically blinks. The muscles of your digestive system also exemplify reflexive action in that they move
food from the stomach to small and large intestines involuntar-
ily. The size of your muscles (the amount of cells they possess)
is determined by your genes. Also determined by your genetic
make-up is the amount of *slow-* and *fast-twitch muscle cells*
you have. Slow-twitch cells predominate during endurance
type of movements and fast-twitch during short bursts of rapid
action, such as is typical of sprinting. Males have more muscle
mass than females, and unfortunately, aging takes a toll on
muscle, tendon, and ligament size. But regular exercise, in particular resistance training, can prevent *atrophy* (shrinking of
muscles and connective tissue).

Skeletal muscle is the basis for exercise and requires energy in order to contract. This energy is in chemical form and is actually contained in the muscle cell itself. However, after short periods of time, this fuel is depleted and unless it is replaced, the muscle fatigues and can no longer contract. This is where nutritional factors enter the picture. I'll discuss diet in Chapter 6 and explain how your eating habits are very much related to your capacity to perform physical activity.

How Exercise Influences the Body's Systems

So much for our brief review. It's also necessary that you appreciate the ways in which the different systems interact with exercise. Earlier in this chapter you were introduced to the concepts of exercise and fitness. You understand that their meanings are intertwined, but that there are distinctions between them. Let's now see how exercise and these systems operate in partnership.

THE OXYGEN REQUIREMENT

Oxygen fuels the body's cells. Without it they die. You are able to store a limited amount of this essential gas in certain depots in the body. But because exercise requires so much of this valuable commodity, the supply is rather quickly depleted. During exercise the replacement process should be ongoing and involve reintroduction of substantial amounts of oxygen. This is even true while participating in anaerobic activities. When swimming under water, for example, after a minute or two, the powerful urge to surface and bring in air cannot be denied. In fact, the brain's breathing center sends "emergency" signals that compel you to come up for a bite of environmental air. Inadequate circulation of blood or insufficient supplies of it are serious deterrents to exercise. The blood is the ultimate repository of oxygen, and the circulatory system energized by the pumping heart is tasked with its distribution.

All efforts of the body's cells produce waste materials that must be expelled. Just as you relieve yourself of the byproducts of digested food, so must each animal cell be rid of the carbon dioxide that results from its metabolism (check the explanations of the terms *metabolism* and *carbon dioxide* that are provided previously in this chapter). This waste gas is dumped into the circulating blood and carried to the lungs. It is then expelled via the process of *exhalation* (the reverse of *inhalation*, or bring environmental air in to the body). "Dirty" air is thus blown away. This discharge of carbon dioxide is also very much a part of the process known as *respiration*, which involves more than merely bringing air into the lungs. Although blood circulation is not the exclusive means of ridding the body of metabolic waste products, it plays an essential role in the excretion of the gas carbon dioxide. When this gas is for some reason not expelled efficiently, its accumulation contributes to the sensation of *fatigue*, which is often a result of engagement in rigorous physical activity. However, the good news is that *training* (explained in this chapter) typically results in more efficient respiration, as well as a more conservative use of oxygen. So as you continue to exercise (wisely and properly), you are expected to improve upon the manner in which you bring in air from the environment, use it, and get rid of the gaseous waste products of cellular activity.

If a theme or bottom line exists in this chapter, it is that *exercise strengthens your body's biological systems*. After extended participation in a program that is sound and well conceived, your systems become more efficient and capable. For instance, the heartbeat will eventually become stronger and pump a greater volume of blood with each contraction. (This is what is meant by efficiency: more output, less effort.) Continued participation should also result in higher concentrations of oxygen in the blood and the removal of gaseous waste products, delaying the onset of muscle fatigue. Another positive outcome is a more competent nervous system that is more capable of processing information and issuing important sensory and motor signals to all systems. All individuals may benefit in these ways, irrespective of age, degree of involvement in exercise, type of exercise, or physical and mental limitations. Although some disabilities impose certain restrictions in movement, exercise has something beneficial for everyone.

Older Adulthood, Exercise, and Physical Well-Being

Your body organs are part of evolved biological systems. Your lungs belong to the respiratory system; the heart, to the circulatory system; the liver, to the digestive system; and your bones, to the skeletal system. Most systems respond very favorably to physical training and during weeks, and months of regular and strategic lifting, moving, bending, stretching, huffing and puffing, they improve in the way they discharge their responsibilities. They become stronger, have more endurance, and generally operate with greater efficiency. Your daily efforts in the vegetable garden, your regular walks, swims, or jogs become easier because the large muscles that account for body movement have undergone change. In addition, your circulatory system is better able to transport oxygen and nutrients throughout your body.

On the other hand, as you age your body becomes increasingly less efficient at converting oxygen into energy. But once again exercise is the savior. It retards this decline. This benefit may be expected no matter your age, although exercisers in their teens, 20s, and 30s will respond to regular exercise more dramatically because they are advantaged by their particular hormonal situation. Aging is associated with a decrease in many kinds of hormone production, including those that stimulate muscle growth. But once again, exercise serves to slow down this decrease and despite your having passed through the teenage years a long time ago, you can benefit muscularly from exercise.

Irrespective of age, as the functional abilities of your organs and systems improve due to exercise, your level of comfort in executing daily physical tasks also improves. Lifting and reaching for things become easier, as does breathing during physical activities that are not necessarily thought of as being of the exercise variety. Therefore, you depend less and less on other persons to do things for you. You require less assistance and attain higher levels of self-confidence and independence. As your muscles become stronger and your joints more flexible, your appearance is also likely to change. What was once a hassle to achieve is now easy or easier to accomplish.

PSYCHOSOCIAL EFFECTS OF EXERCISE

A number of years ago one of my doctoral students, Kathy Gill, devised a study in conjunction with her dissertation research that used older persons as participants. The average age of her male and female subjects was about 80 years. Kathy required her subjects to participate in a regular and supervised walking program. She arranged for them to be transported by van to a nearby park where they walked for 45 minutes over a period of 10 weeks under her supervision.

Although it was necessary for some participants to use canes or walkers, all were nonetheless asked to proceed with the walk to their best ability. Another group did not exercise but played backgammon under Kathy's supervision for the same amount of minutes and days per week.

Prior to beginning their program of exercise, participants were tested with paper and pencil inventories that probed their perceptions about "hassles" (things in their life that regularly seemed difficult). Examples of hassles in this case were dressing, tying shoe laces, and reaching for canned food on a high pantry shelf. Assorted social factors, which involved troublesome interactions with others (neighbors, relatives, etc.), were additionally included in the scale. Men and women in the study also answered questions on other scales that examined their perceptions about general quality of life, frequency of stressful experiences, and distressing physical symptoms.

Participants were led to believe that the study's essential purpose was to determine to what extent their physical fitness might have been altered as a result of the exercise regimen. No mention was made of Kathy's real interest: the potential effects of the walking program upon the psychosocial status of subjects.

At the conclusion of the program, participants again answered questions on the various inventories. What Kathy's findings revealed was a very marked change in reported perceptions about hassles, stressors, and physical symptoms, all in favorable directions. When you undertake a regular program of exercise and stick with it, your entire outlook about yourself and how you function in your personal world, how you think of yourself and how you deal with others, changes for the better. Or at least, these things stand a very good chance of changing for the better.

BODY FAT AND EXERCISE

Aging tends to bring with it a tendency for a greater percentage of your body weight to be fat. Trousers and sport coats button more snuggly. Buttocks, thighs, and hips require more space in skirts and jeans. Exercise can inhibit this tendency. Now here's the skinny (pun intended) on fat.

You store two kinds of fat: *subcutaneous* and *visceral*. The former is found beneath your skin, and you are very much aware of its presence. When you evaluate an acquaintance as being chubby or too heavy, your judgment is based upon what you see. And what you see and react to is that person's subcutaneous fat. A certain amount of this material is essential for good health. Among other things, it keeps you warm. It also accounts in large measure for your body's shape. Fat is not bad. But excess fat is.

Visceral fat is internal fat and covers and protects your internal organs. It's not really obvious how much of this material you actually have. Magnetic resonance imaging (MRI) is an approved method for determining your exact quantity. However, the amount of both kinds of stored fat correlates with the amount of exercise you do as well as your caloric intake. If the caloric intake is greater than what your tissues, organs, and systems need to function healthfully, the leftover calories will be stored as fat, both subcutaneous and visceral.

Barring certain metabolic disorders that affect some persons, this concept of caloric or energy balance, referred to by scientists as *thermodynamics*, is pretty straightforward. Larger than necessary amounts of stored visceral fat are associated with heart and blood vessel disease, hypertension (high blood pressure), diabetes mellitus, and arthritis. As you age beyond your 60s and 70s, the likelihood of having one or more of these conditions increases irrespective of the amount of visceral and subcutaneous fat you have. However, exercise will increase the degree to which body fat is metabolized or burned up. Your stored body fat is an important fuel for muscular function—not the exclusive fuel, but a very vital one. Therefore, the more you exercise (again, sensibly and safely), the more fat you burn. The more you burn, the less fat you store, and the logical conclusion is that you are thus less likely to develop cardiovascular disease, diabetes, and high blood pressure.

However, a caveat is in order here. I admit to being biased in presenting a case for programmatic physical activity. Throughout this book I argue repeatedly in favor of exercise for all, but particularly for Boomers and those who are older. Thematically, this is what the book is all about. Having read but a few pages of this chapter you certainly realize where I stand. Now, here's the caveat: *It takes an awful lot of exercise to significantly reduce your stored body fat.*

My hope is that all readers of this book will undertake a strategic and regular exercise program. However, if meaningful reduction of body fat is your goal, certainly a legitimate one at that, your job will be formidable if increased physical activity is your exclusive modus operandi. To lose weight, reducing your caloric intake in tandem with physical activity is preferred. Without reducing calorie intake, you'd have to jog more than 20 miles to lose a single pound of stored body fat, certainly an inefficient approach to regulating body weight.

But don't misinterpret my point. Exercise will help, but you'll have to do more than merely increasing your physical activity, unless you are prepared to wait a very long time for the needle on your bathroom scale to move in a gratifying direction. Over the long run, those who run exceptionally long distances will eventually slim down. And those 20 or more miles that have to be logged in order to lose a pound of stored fat need not be done in one shot. A *cumulative effect* is possible, collecting this distance over a period of time. In other words you can account for that one pound if you jog one mile a day for 20 days (if caloric intake is kept constant). You can do it this way, but you had better have an awful lot of patience at your disposal, because we're talking about a 20-day effort for a loss of only one pound of fat. Most folks who desire to lose weight are interested in much more than one pound.

A few more points about stored body fat: You can't get rid of it precisely where you wish. You can't spot reduce fat. You can do a thousand sit-ups daily and still not say goodbye to your love handles, per se. What you can do through exercise in combination with dietary regulation is reduce your total amount of stored body fat by burning calories with the hope that the area you've targeted indeed yields what you desire. We tend to store subcutaneous fat in very personal ways and locations. In some of us storage occurs in the hips, neck, face, or thigh areas. In others, fat tends to collect elsewhere. Look for a more detailed discussion of fat storage in Chapter 3. I'll briefly reiterate some of these notions about stored fat and discuss additional aspects, notably a popular and convenient but problematic method of determining how fat you are, namely the *body mass index*.

EXERCISE AND THE IMMUNE SYSTEM

I've already referred to the way in which we think of our body organs as being arranged in systems. I mentioned the respiratory, digestive, and circulatory systems. One other very important physiological system should be added to the list, namely the *immune system*, whose mandate it is to attack any potentially harmful substance that invades your body. Essentially, your immune system is designed to protect you from destructive microorganisms or poisons that in some way compromise your health. Snake venom would be one example; an infection of some sort would be another. There are different varieties of these protective cells, one of which is the white blood cell, although your immune system has other defensive components that interact in complex ways, I'll restrict our discussion to the white blood cell.

Scattered abundantly throughout your body are lymph nodes where different kinds of white corpuscles are stored. When trouble looms, such as the presence of harmful bacteria, these corpuscles are rushed to the site of bacterial invasion via a network of tubules akin to those in the circulatory system. If you have a throat infection you can feel the swollen lymph nodes in your neck laden with white corpuscles. The nodes in your groin similarly enlarge when an infection is brewing in your abdominal area or thigh. The invading organisms are surrounded and devoured by the white blood cells (called white because they are colorless).

Needless to say, the protection offered by your immune system is vital, but unfortunately, as we age, the potency of this private battalion of dedicated warriors is compromised. Perhaps you've noticed a few more colds or sore throats annually than in your earlier years. I know such comparisons are difficult to make because many factors contribute to the onset of a throat infection or common cold.

However, aging does reduce immune system strength. Your physician, if he or she is like mine, therefore makes a yearly appeal for you to sign up for flu shots and other preemptive and precautionary injections. The good news is that exercise can also strengthen your immune system and restore some of its age-related lost vitality. But the exercise should not be highly intense if the objective is to strengthen the immune system. Too much stress on the body will affect the immune system adversely. Moderate physical activity will provide best results. You've got to support the efforts of these defenders who are ready to serve with your help.

Here's the guiding principle: *moderate exercise boosts the immune system; intense exercise has the opposite effect.* As your body responds to exercise, the protective immune cells circulate more quickly and are therefore better able to destroy viruses and bacteria. In a few hours after moderate exercise the immune system returns to normal levels. A program of regular exercise will maintain higher levels for a more extended time. That's why moderately strenuous physical activity, done on a regular basis, is the key to better overall immunity. The immune system also needs time to recover, so it's important to build in rest days in your activity schedule, particularly if you become involved in distance walking, running, or swimming.

BENEFICIAL EFFECTS OF EXERCISE ON THE IMMUNE SYSTEM—HOW THEY WORK

Exactly how and why does exercise affect the immune system? It seems that the contraction and relaxation of the skeletal muscles during limb and body movement, in combination with an increase in volume and rate of breathing—typical reactions to exercise—trigger increased lymph node activity. With an abundance of white cells available when needed, you get a higher level of protection against invading and potentially harmful agents.

PROTEIN, EXERCISE, AND THE IMMUNE SYSTEM

Exercise, particularly resistance exercise (weight training, for example), results in increased muscle mass. The more muscle mass in the body, the more protein in the body. The more protein in your body, the more protein available in reserve for use in immune system operations when necessary (when an additional supply of white blood cell is suddenly needed). Protein is an essential ingredient for white blood cell production. However, too much exercise may consume this abundant supply of reserve protein because your muscles will require extra amounts for their repair and maintenance. Thus less protein is available for immune system function. Therefore, once again, don't be too ambitious with your exercise: don't overdo it if you have the best interest of your immune system in mind. But be mindful that another benefit of a sensible, properly designed program of regular exercise is strengthening of the immune system. But realize that in addition, nutritional factors also influence your immune system's ability to do its job. I'll have more to say about nutrition in Chapter 3.

CORTISOL AND EXERCISE

Specialized cells in your body manufacture chemical products known as *hormones*. They are delivered directly into the bloodstream via special ducts or tubes, which results in very rapid

distribution. One such hormone is *cortisol,* whose blood level is
elevated during times of stress and anxiety. The higher the concentration of this hormone in your blood, the higher your stress
response. Your feeling of discomfort during stress and anxiety
is due in part to elevation of cortisol. The nervous system picks
up on this increase in hormonal concentration and sends messages to your brain that you interpret as distress. One way in
which scientists can ascertain a stress reaction, be it physical or
psychological, is to assess blood cortisol levels. In Chapter 6 I'll
elaborate upon this physiological linkage further.

Unlike other hormones that decrease with aging, cortisol levels remain pretty much the same well into your 60s and beyond.
People our age maintain levels comparable to when we were
much younger, but these levels fluctuate during the day, depending upon stress. Exercise can burn off undesirably high
concentrations of cortisol and thereby reduce stress-related discomfort (distress). It's important, however, to return to the caution I provided earlier: Exercise that is too vigorous can result in
the opposite effect. Intense exercise is likely to elevate cortisol
levels. Moderation is the keynote, and for this reason, as you
make your way through this book, you'll continue to read about
the importance of sensible, well-designed programs of physical
activity. By all means, exercise but don't overdo it.

Along these lines is yet another documented physical or
physiological benefit of participation in regular exercise for
older persons. Researchers at The Ohio State University have
reported that the wounds of older individuals who are fit heal
more quickly than those of sedentary persons. And the faster a
wound heals, the less the risk of it becoming infected. A lower
incidence of infection means less work for your immune system—it gets a break. The white blood cells are thus saved for
when they are really needed. Another pay-off of exercise!

EXERCISE AND THE SKIN

The skin is an organ—and the body's largest organ at that. You
may have never thought of this highly visible layer of protective material that covers the body as such. Your skin accounts

for approximately one-seventh of your entire body weight and serves as a protective barrier against potentially harmful organisms or any other agents seeking to infiltrate your body. Unfortunately, the anti-aging effects of exercise upon the skin have not received much attention even by those who promote regular exercise. But this connection exists. Your skeletal muscles and cardiorespiratory mechanisms are not the only beneficiaries of exercise.

As you age, your skin changes. Its elastic quality gradually diminishes; it becomes thinner and retains less moisture. Aging skin also heals more slowly after being cut or burned. Many of these changes are due to sun exposure. In particular is the appearance on older persons of brown spots and wrinkles. Although the sun is usually the culprit in skin changes, even skin that has been protected with clothing or sunscreen over the years will age, but much less dramatically. The term *photoaging* refers to changes in the skin due to long-term sun exposure. *Intrinsic aging* on the other hand, refers to changes due to nothing more than the passage of many years.

First, realize that regular exercise is usually associated with sweating, which is helpful in unclogging pores in the skin and therefore providing a cleansing or detoxifying effect. Second, during exercise the circulation of blood increases throughout the body, including the skin. Thus, skin cells are saturated with oxygen and other nutrients, particularly those that enhance the production of *collagen* (a form of connective tissue that plumps up your skin, reduces formation of wrinkles, and enables the face to have a youthful appearance).

The better your circulation, the more effective your natural skin cleansing process. Exercise definitely improves circulatory function. Drinking plenty of water during exercise will improve blood flow to the skin. Forget about special facial exercises. Dermatologists tell us that they are a waste of time and may even increase the appearance of wrinkles and lines. Consider using total body exercise as a strategy if your aim is healthier skin.

Collagen production tends to decease during aging, resulting in drier and more wrinkled skin, but exercise can interfere with this deterioration. This is why those who exercise generally have better overall complexions. Persons with certain existing skin diseases may find that exercise aggravates these conditions. But for most of us exercise truly helps. When exercising out of doors, sunglasses and a cap or head-covering of some sort are absolutely necessary. If you are swimming, a brimmed cap or sunglasses are not practical (although tinted goggles are a distinct possibility). However, sunscreen should definitely be applied prior to pool entry and replenished on the skin from time to time because the stuff will wear off during an extended workout. Use sunscreen with a sun protection factor (SPF) of 15 or higher. *Wear protective head and body coverings to prevent sunrays from counteracting the benefits of exercise to the skin.*

Outdoor heat generated by the sun may increase stress levels during exercise. Older individuals may have diminished internal heat regulation mechanisms that are activated in order to adjust for rising body temperature. Heat regulation is a function of a specific brain center—the *hypothalamus*—and is reflexive or automatic. When you are hot, you sweat; when very cold, you shiver. No cognition is involved. Out of doors exercise should be done early in the morning before the sun is high, or in the evening after it has gone down. Your personal lifestyle, circadian rhythms, and preferences all can help you determine when to exercise. My preference has always been for early morning.

I've been praising the many healthful psychological and physical benefits of exercise in this chapter, and I have one more to add, or rather, a potential benefit. Findings from recent research done with mice and rats enable the speculation that exercise offers protection against two kinds of cancer: skin and colon cancer (actually precancerous polyps in the intestine as well as malignant tumors). Certainly, there's a world of difference between humans and rodents. Moreover, the reasons for such links with exercise have not yet been definitively determined, although the authors of these studies provide some very plausible explanations. And of course, the available studies showing a reduction of certain kinds of cancer in the face of regular physical activity are not without their critics. (I'll have additional comments about the association between cancer and exercise in Chapter 2.)

At any rate, there's no denying that many advances in medical science that have enormously advantaged humans began with animal studies, particularly advances that deal with cancer. And I say this with sincere deference to my many friends who are animal rights devotees. The mouse studies that I'm referring to are about four or five years old, but it would not surprise me if by the time this book made its way into your hands, additional research with human subjects that verifies the animal findings will have been conducted. Time will tell. Although a rodent is a far cry from what's transpiring in our human bodies, findings from mouse and rat research do provide ideas and models that enable scientists to understand our physiological phenomena. Some such recent studies suggest that exercise has a counteracting effect upon skin cancer in mice. It appears to stimulate the destruction of developing tumors' biology. In this way, exercise actually protects the skin, and exercisers have lower incidences of skin cancer than sedentary persons.

Falling and Exercise

Falling can be a life-changing event for Boomers and older adults. Unfortunately, falling is all too common within these populations. Close to 14,000 men and women 65 and older die from fall-related injuries each year in the United States alone. This boils down to the impressive and alarming figure of about one person per hour. Of these, more than 60% are 75 and older. Older women in particular and the elderly living alone are likely to fall, as are frail individuals, those with poor vision, or people who have gait and balance problems. Each year, one-third of the population 65 years and older experiences at least one fall, and half of those fall repeatedly.[5]

Those with low strength levels and little physical activity in their daily lives are twice as likely to fall as healthier people of the same age. And when older persons with the above deficits do fall, they sustain relatively more severe injuries. Falls are the most common cause of hospital admissions for trauma, and in most, or at least many, cases can be entirely avoided. Even if a fall doesn't result in fatality or serious injury, it may exert a negative influence on your life. Decreased self confidence, fear of falling again, and curtailment of activities that involve locomotion may be consequences that reduce the quality of life.

Balance is a *neuromuscular* action, meaning that your central nervous system relays messages to your connective tissue and muscles about contracting and relaxing. This is what accounts for your maintenance of equilibrium and upright position in space. Some of these messages originate in the middle ear, others in your brain itself. We wage unrelenting battle with one of nature's most powerful forces, the force of gravity, which stubbornly strives to pull us down. Fortunately, special *antigravity muscles* located, among other places, in your back, keep flexing and relaxing in critical sequences. They are monitored and controlled by the nervous system in a valiant attempt to keep you upright. This sequential action is automatic and therefore requires no conscious effort. You don't have to think about these things. You simply go about your day while these protective mechanisms operate on your behalf.

But if these antigravity muscles are weak, or for any reason they are unprepared to meet their obligations, you're in for trouble. As we age these autonomic procedures do weaken somewhat and a bit of their effectiveness is lost. Put a little more bluntly, as we get older our ability to sustain balance weakens and we are vulnerable to tipping over when changes in our physical environment suddenly occur. Just as muscles all throughout the body tend to atrophy during aging, these so-called balance muscles (antigravity muscles) also weaken over the years. To boot, an elderly skeletal system is not what it was during youth and early adulthood. A considerable amount of bone density has been lost and a heavy fall may therefore take a greater toll on your bones, which are more susceptible to breaking.

So what's the connection between falling and exercise? You can anticipate my answer. Participation in regular exercise eventually improves and strengthens neuromuscular communication—or at least retards its deterioration. You'll not succeed in reversing age-related changes in any of your body systems, but exercise will slow them down or enable you to maintain a much more steady level of systemic health. In other words, through exercise you can flatten out the graph depicting negative change. Long-term exercise involving weight-bearing movements, such as walking or dancing, tends to increase the density of your bones (number of bone cells in your limbs). Higher bone density means more strength and durability, which in turn means greater resistance to fracture.

An additional point about balance: Don't think about it as a general ability. A good analogy would be intelligence. It's improper to talk about a person being very intelligent because there are various kinds of intelligence. A person can be strong in mathematical ability and very weak in the ability to use language effectively. Some psychologists enumerate as many as eight intelligences, such as spatial, interpersonal (getting along with others), musical, bodily kinesthetic (handling objects skillfully and controlling one's body in space), linguistic (facility in acquiring alternative language), logical, mathematical (facility in grasping mathematical concepts), and naturalistic (understanding phenomena occurring in nature). We vary with regard to the strength of these different kinds of intelligence, and few of us are very high or very low in all of them. This suggests that when describing a person's intelligence, it is necessary to be specific about the particular intellectual ability in question.

The very same notion should be applied to balance. Because different kinds of balance exist, it is incorrect to say, for instance, that "She has great balance" or "His balance is weak." Is the balancing requirement for the circus tightrope artist the same as for the water skier or ballet dancer? Of course not. Some activities emphasize holding a certain position while the body is stationary. Others demand maintenance of the upright position while moving in space (snow skiing). All forms of balance are responsive to training, training that involves the nervous and muscular systems. By strengthening the neuromuscular connections and working to improve the functional abilities of balance muscles through exercise, you can improve the chances of resisting falling when caught off guard by a bathroom wet spot or uneven bedroom carpet.

Another possible cause of falling in the Boomer years and beyond is debilitated vision. Let me therefore offer a brief remark as an addendum to our discussion of falling. As our visual capabilities change so may the clarity with which we receive certain stimuli from the environment that are instrumental in maintaining balance. We are always processing information about characteristics of our surroundings such as distance, depth, and height. We receive information about these factors and make judgments and decisions about the ways in which we move or position ourselves in the physical environment based upon this input. If and when the incoming data are insufficient, distorted, or not forthcoming, our ability to move or maintain equilibrium is challenged or reduced.

Imagine waking up one morning and feeling different—more

THE BENEFITS OF DAILY PHYSICAL ACTIVITY
Source: American Heart Association

- Reduces the risk of heart disease
- Keeps weight under control
- Improves cholesterol levels
- Prevents and manages high blood pressure
- Prevents bone loss
- Boosts energy levels
- Helps manage stress
- Releases tension
- Improves the ability to fall asleep quickly and sleep well
- Improves self-image
- Counters anxiety and depression
- Increases enthusiasm and optimism

- Enhances muscle strength, increasing the ability to do other physical activities
- Provides a way to share an activity with family and friends
- Establishes good heart-healthy habits in children and counters the conditions that lead to heart attack and stroke later in life, including obesity, high blood pressure, poor cholesterol levels, and poor lifestyle habits
- Delays or prevents chronic illnesses and diseases associated with aging
- Maintains quality of life and independence longer

vibrant and better prepared for the day than ever before. Over the long run exercise can generate such a feeling.

☞ WHAT YOU'VE LEARNED IN THIS CHAPTER

This chapter was intended to encourage you to get going on an exercise program despite your age and possible history of limited participation in regular physical activity. Two themes were implicit: 1) It is never too late to get started, and 2) Older men and women, in particular, can benefit significantly from exercise—in fact, more so than any other age group.

Deterioration of certain mental abilities is slower in exercisers who are 60 and older in comparison to sedentary persons. Higher levels of circulatory and nervous system health and vitality derived from fitness are likely the reason. Perceptions of depression and fatigue decrease right after a bout of exercise, and short-term improvements in self-concept, body image, and happiness may be anticipated after a workout. These psychological factors are critical parts of your makeup and their modification in positive directions can only contribute to your total mental health picture.

In this section you also learned about fat storage: the beneficial role it plays in your body as well as the association of excess storage with high blood pressure, diabetes, and arthritis. The manner in which exercise helps regulate the amount of stored body fat was clarified.

You also learned about immune function. Designed to protect your body from harmful invading organisms, this system, and the white blood cells it produces, is strengthened by regular exercise done at appropriate levels of intensity. However, inappropriate amounts and intensities of exercise may exert an opposite effect. Wounds of older persons heal more rapidly when their fitness levels are high because of exercise.

You also learned about the ways in which your skin, the body's largest organ, is benefited by exercise; how strong circulation associated with high levels of fitness provides for relatively better skin cleansing. And that the incidence of skin cancer is found to be lower among elderly persons who exercise.

Falling, a bane to older persons, is the last subject addressed in this chapter. Weight-bearing exercise contributes to higher density in your body's bones, which helps them resist fracture if and when a fall occurs. The probability of losing balance and falling is reduced when you achieve high levels of fitness. By strengthening muscle groups that have primary responsibility for maintaining balance and counteracting the force of gravity, the likelihood of falling can be reduced.

FOOD FOR THOUGHT

1	Have you ever noticed that during or right after exercise, facts and recollections that you tried in vain to retrieve earlier suddenly became available? Speculate as to why this happened.
2	Do you consider your lifestyle to be active? What criteria would you apply to determine that your lifestyle is too active or not active enough?
3	What views do you have about the shape of your body? Are you pleased with it? Is it in need modification? Are you prepared to take steps that might lead to a reconfiguration of your body shape?
4	Have you thought about how to take a fall? Do you know how to go down safely when and if you fall? Specifically, what would you do if you felt yourself losing control of your upright position?

Endnotes

1. January 9, 2011, p. 14.
2. Marcus, Mary Brophy. *USA Today*, July 12, 2010.
3. June 24, 2008.
4. March 2, 2010.
5. Trombetti, Hars, Hermann, et al., 2010

Chapter 2

Exercise, Wellness, Health, and Illness

Your physician gives you a clean bill of health and reports that "you're healthy as a horse and fit as a fiddle." Why these similes? Don't horses get sick? They can't be healthy all of the time. And what's so terrific about having the fitness level of a violin? What have violins to do with strong and organically sound human bodies? But since you've apparently passed every laboratory and office test with flying colors, you interpret the doctor's remark as good news. Not a troublesome finding in his entire report. But something is troubling you. You don't feel particularly healthy despite the physician's report. Could there be another vital health component beyond serum cholesterol, blood sugar, blood pressure, heart rate, and prostate-specific antigen (PSA—if you're male)? Is there another aspect of your health that the doctor may have missed? Maybe you enjoy good health. But what about your wellness? Perhaps your physician doesn't deal with wellness.

What is *wellness*? Is it different than *health*? Is it measurable? Can you be *healthy* but not *well*? Is it possible that despite favorable results from lab tests, you are still unwell? How does the concept of *illness* enter the picture? Is it different from wellness and health? And how do these matters relate to exercise?

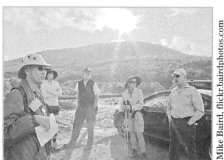

Mike Baird, flickr.bairdphotos.com

Wellness and health, while similar, aren't necessarily the same. Despite an increasingly failing heart or rampant cancer that may be getting the best of you, you can still enjoy a high degree of wellness.

Health and illness are intertwined concepts. If your health is poor, you are ill because health is contingent upon soundness of biological organs and systems. This is what the term health means. When all systems are go, you are healthy. When disease or trauma undermines your biological processes or when infection interferes with the function of your organs, you are ill. But health is more than the absence of illness, although the two exist in an intimate relationship. As one goes up, the other goes down. When your illness is low, you're in good health.

As you mull over these contrasts, realize that barring a medical diagnosis of imminent demise, not all of your vital systems necessarily fail or become faulty simultaneously. They do so over time. Your automobile's transmission, brakes, air conditioning, and engine do not fail in synchrony unless the machine is driven off a cliff and shattered. The same is true of your body's systems. Your digestive system may be seriously compromised, but your circulatory mechanisms could remain perfectly strong and functional in every respect. Your vision may be weakened, but your nervous system may remain entirely intact and properly functional.

Table 2.1. Wellness, Health, Illness and Fitness—In Comparison			
Wellness	**Health**	**Illness**	**Fitness**
Everything in balance	*Organic soundness*	*Systemic organic malfunction*	*Prepared to meet daily demands*
components	spiritual emotional physical mental social	All systems are "go"	Disease, infection	Depends on your work and require- ments imposed by daily activities

Wellness is different. Despite an increasingly failing heart or rampant cancer that may be getting the best of you, you can still enjoy a high degree of wellness. Even very ill persons under the threat of impending death may score high on wellness because wellness has little to do with illness. Some years ago a friend and former colleague, Dr. Jerrold Greenberg, and I made these distinctions in a book we collaborated upon (*Physical Fitness: A Wellness Approach*). We argued that wellness involves your perception of a satisfactory balance among the important dimensions of your life. When all your psychological and physical ducks are in a neat and secure row; when you know that you are safe, loved, adjusted to life's travails and necessities; when you believe that you are in control of your emotions, doing your best in view of prevailing circumstances, then you enjoy substantial wellness irrespective of prevailing illness.

Try This

Bring to mind a circle or actually draw one on a piece of paper. Fill the circle with words or terms that represent characteristics of your physical and psychological selves. By this I mean attributes that surely describe you; your social connections;

your views about your various emotional tendencies (anger easily, compassionate, etc.) Your circle should be absolutely round and unbroken. If not, the definition of circle is unsatisfied.

Next, convert this imaginary circle to a wheel with spokes that divide it into segments. Let each segment represent one category of yourself. For instance, let one segment be devoted to your mental status, another to your social efforts and achievements, and another to your spiritual endeavors. Find a place for all the physical, social, and psychological attributes that you've located in the circle.

Now imagine that one of the wheel's components is problematic. For instance, the segment that represents your interpersonal relations. Perhaps you have few acquaintances and no true friends. Thus a bump or rough spot mars your wheel, making its roundness imperfect. It becomes less smooth and its capacity to roll smoothly is compromised. Your wellness is thus diminished.

If this one aspect of the circle is all that is troublesome, then you're okay. Your circle or wheel is still able to move forward. But for each bump on the wheel, more and more smoothness is sacrificed. Your life is less round and efficient, and your wellness level increasingly lowers. The wheel knocks and jolts like a flat tire. It flops and yaws and waggles ungracefully in its struggles to advance.

Think of this attempt to move forward as life itself. With a low level of wellness your wheel is able to roll, but its parts are not efficiently integrated nor proportionally developed. The segments are too uneven and unequal. Assume for the moment that your circle or wheel's social dimension is small and underdeveloped in contrast to your exaggerated intellectual segment. This is what I meant in the introduction to this chapter that something that is missing.

YOUR WHEEL OF LIFE

Your wheel of life has five sectors: *physical*, *mental*, *emotional*, *social*, and *spiritual*. *Physical* refers to your body and its parts—to what is commonly spoken of as *health status*—what your physician was speaking of when he used the "fit as a fiddle/healthy as a horse" similes. *Mental* refers to your intellectual abilities and your capacities for thinking and learning. *Emotional* brings to mind your feelings and how you understand, deal with, and control them. *Social* makes reference to your abilities relative to interacting with other persons. Lastly, your *spiritual* self is predicated upon your belief in some force that regulates and accounts for the world in which you live. The degree of your investment in this regulatory power, be it God, nature, or a set of scientific principles, is a measure of your spirituality.

The segments of your wheel are unlikely to be exactly equal in size because some parts are naturally more heavily trafficked and more fully advanced than others. You therefore compensate and adjust your daily behavior in order to make the wheel as rounded as possible so that it rolls smoothly and efficiently. When you recognize that certain parts of your circle have deficiencies or rough spots, or that some are disproportionally thick while others are too thin, you try to improve the situation by altering the dimensions of the improperly sized segments. If one sector is woefully out of kilter, adjustments become difficult and your wheel wobbles and falters. Your overall wellness decreases proportionally.

Are you now able to see how it's possible to be well despite having one dimension of your life-wheel swollen and uneven or thin and undernourished? If your compensations and adjustments are effective despite initial under- or overdevelopment of some sectors of the wheel, your roll will be nice, and life will be delightful. You'll be well. You can buy that shirt you saw hanging in the t-shirt shop in the mall that says "Life is good." You can saunter about displaying it with conviction. The important point to bear in mind is that you can be healthy (disease free) but not very well. And you can be ill but very well (suffering from a serious malady, but wheel sectors are nicely balanced and supportive of one another).

IMBALANCES AMONG WHEEL SEGMENTS

If you ignore one or more segments of the circle and your adjustments are inadequate, your level of wellness continues to depreciate. Though your physical component might be whole-some, if your social or emotional dimensions are weak and flac-cid, your wellness is low. Ideally, you are looking for a nicely balanced wheel with all your sectors mutually supportiver de-spite their inequality in size. You are seeking to establish mu-tual support among wheel segments.

EXERCISE, HEALTH, WELLNESS, AND ILLNESS: LINKS AND ISSUES

In Chapter 1, I defined the term *exercise* as "rigorous physical activity done with the aim of improving some aspect of physi-cal fitness." Your fitness status depends on your ability to sat-isfy the specific physical demands that you encounter on a daily basis. Fitness can be assessed through various standard-ized physical tests. This is not the case with wellness. Relevant questions must be asked and answered to determine how well you are. Answers must be given honestly if you or the profes-sional posing the questions on your behalf is to capture a rea-sonably clear and helpful picture of your wellness wheel. In or-der to get a grip on your wellness status, you must be prepared to write or talk about all five of the wheel's components as they relate to your life.

A BIT MORE ABOUT EXERCISE AND FITNESS

Bear in mind that exercise is more than physical activity. If an activity is to be considered an authentic exercise, its purpose is physical improvement of some kind. It must be dedicated to a positive change in your strength, endurance, agility, and flexi-bility. Crocheting is a wonderful recreational activity as are contract bridge and chess. But the goal of physical betterment is lacking. One other point: If you are to benefit from exercise *it must be done with regularity and should involve action of large skeletal muscles.*

When contemplating your fitness status or appropriate exer-cise goals, first ask yourself, "Fitness for what? Your fitness is highly specific to your personal goals, common practices, and aspirations. (We'll talk in more depth about setting exercise goals in Chapter 8.) Because all of us differ in how we spend our days and lives, our fitness objectives are understandably not the same. Your ideal fitness target is not the same as that of the collegiate athlete, the mail carrier, the ballerina, the fire-fighter, the seamstress, the butcher, or the next door neighbor.

Although it's possible we would all hold the very same fitness objectives, it's highly unlikely. Most fitness goals are highly specific to an individual: that is, to you. Your fitness goals are yours alone. They are specific to your own personal needs, interests, health, and wellness. The more you and I share personal characteristics, needs, and interests, the more overlap our fitness goals would be likely to have.

If we were all butchers who stood on our feet seven hours each day, slicing and packaging meat, then we would share a major fitness objective: muscular endurance (legs, shoulders, forearms, etc.). We are not all butchers but you and I do have in common our age range. However, even this shared attribute doesn't suggest that our fitness objectives are identical since we all have so many other divergent qualities. Some of us are male, others female. Some of us are employed, and some are retired. Some are single, some married. It stands to reason, therefore, that our fitness goals should also vary widely. Still, irrespective of our differences, we all must address the same *categories of fitness*: muscular strength and endurance, flexibility, agility, and aerobic capacity. *We must pursue the same fitness components, but to different degrees.*

The relationships among fitness, health, illness, and wellness are fourfold:

- You can be well, but ill.
- You can be very healthy, but unwell.
- If your health is compromised, a high level of fitness is unlikely.
- If you enjoy a high level of physical fitness then it's likely that you are well and healthy.

Let's have a closer look at each of the above bulleted items and elaborate upon some points made earlier. Once again, we'll use the wheel as a metaphor. If the five dimensions of your wellness wheel are unequal or out of balance then your wellness is impaired or at least reduced. The extent to which you are unwell depends on the extent of inequality among the five parts of the wheel. If one section becomes more able or stronger in order to compensate for the instability or feebleness of another or others, your wellness deficit is minimal. If the compensation is efficient and effective, even though you may still be ill, your wellness can be substantial.

Your physical and mental health may be sound, but for example, if the social segment of your wheel is feeble or underdeveloped with no compensatory support from other sectors (perhaps the spiritual sector), your wellness is in jeopardy.

If your health is impaired over an extended period of time and you are unable to *train* (exercise with rigor and regularity), your physical fitness level will be low unless you modify your response to the question, "Fitness for what?" In other words, if you are no longer a firefighter or butcher but are now involved in volunteer work at the local library or are working on a novel that you've had in mind for years, you may still have at your disposal an appropriate level of fitness to satisfy the demands of your day. Your fitness goals should be reconfigured on a regular basis, particularly when significant health or lifestyle changes occur.

OVERDOING IT

A high level of physical fitness is usually indicative of good health and wellness. However, a very high level of fitness may also be the result of training that has been so intense and unrelenting that it pushes other wheel segments out of equilibrium. The simplest way for me to explain this is with the expression *overdoing*. An obsessive commitment to exercise may yield a high level of fitness, but at the expense of other dimensions of the wellness wheel. You may be neglecting your family, circumventing professional or career requirements, avoiding social obligations, and as I suggest in Chapter 5, setting yourself up for injury.

An exercise topic that attracted me for years is *running ad-*

diction. At one point in my career I devoted considerable time and energy to studying, writing, and lecturing about this phenomenon. I believe I and former graduate student Michael Sachs (now a professor at Temple University) were among the first—if not the very first—to write about it. Michael did his doctoral dissertation on this subject.

Running addiction or dependence is ironically problematic. Those who train with a ferocious commitment, who unfailingly run long distances six or seven days a week, and who suffer pangs of deprivation when unable to do so, fall into this category. Their psychophysiological dependence upon running is so powerful that they permit no obstacle to deprive them of the experience. Like the noble mail carrier, undaunted by sleet, rain, or any other vagaries of weather, this kind of exerciser proceeds in ways that abuse health and wellness. Social relationships suffer. Work effort and on-the-job commitment are compromised and family responsibilities are not given their due. Wellness wheels are distorted and wellness levels remain low despite the runner/jogger's robust respiratory system. It's not likely that elderly persons who are initially embarking upon a jogging or walking regimen would fall prey to this condition. But those of you at the very beginning of Boomerhood (right at 60 years of age or very close to it) just might. Be aware of this possibility despite your momentary conviction that it is an unrealistic eventuality. Be careful of overdoing exercise. *Strive for high levels of health, wellness, and fitness while keeping as low a level of illness as possible.*

Some Common Boomer Medical Issues: How Exercise Can Help

In each phase of your life, certain illnesses or health challenges arise and typify a particular stage of development. Acne is not something that afflicts toddlers, but is certainly a bane to teenagers. High cholesterol values are not usually a concern of preschool children. They do, of course, relate importantly to the health of middle-aged and elderly patients. Ironically, some conditions such as bladder regulation and continence problems

Reducing the probability of some common illnesses and ailments through exercise—or "I love this doctor."

There's a cute, albeit entirely misleading, anecdote circulating on the internet among friends who share what they consider to be amusing health-related stories. I'm sure there's a very large tongue in the capacious cheek of the physician interviewed in this bit of nonsense. His comments are worth sharing if only to reveal their naiveté. I shudder when contemplating the number of exercise deniers who accept this information and are only too pleased to bolster their ill-conceived defense of physical inactivity and poor eating habits. The piece is titled "I love this doctor." Enjoy it but don't take it too seriously.

Q: Doctor, I've heard that cardiovascular exercise can prolong life. Is this true?

A: The heart is only good for so many beats, so don't waste any on exercise. Everything wears out eventually. Speeding up your heart rate does not make you live longer; which is like saying you can extend the life of your car by driving faster. If you want to live longer take a nap.

Q: Should I cut down on meat and eat more fruits and vegetables?

A: You must grasp the logistical implications for efficiency here. What does a cow eat? Hay and corn. What are these? Vegetables. So steak is nothing more than an efficient mechanism for delivering vegetables to your system. Does your body require grain? Eat chicken. Beef is also a good source of field grass (green leafy vegetable). And pork chops can provide 100% recommended daily allowance of vegetable products.

Q: Should I reduce my alcohol intake?

A: No, not at all. Wine is made from fruit. Brandy is distilled wine. That means that water is removed from fruit, which means that you derive even more benefit. Beer is also made out of grain. So, bottoms up!

Q: How can I calculate my body/fat ration?

A: If you have a body and you have fat, the ratio is one to one. If you have two bodies, the ratio is two to one, etc.

Q: What are some of the advantages of participating in a regular exercise program?

A: I cannot think of a single one. Sorry. My philosophy is: No pain . . . good.

Q: Aren't fried foods bad for you?

A: You aren't listening! Fried foods are fried in vegetable oil. How can getting more vegetables be bad for you?

Q: Will sit-ups help prevent me from getting a little soft around the middle?

A: Definitely not! When you exercise a muscle, it gets bigger. You should only do sit-ups if you want a bigger stomach.

Q: Is chocolate bad for me?

A: Are you crazy? HELLO . . . The cocoa bean is a vegetable! And it is the best feel-good food around.

Q: Is swimming good for your figure?

A: If swimming is good for your figure, explain whales to me.

Q: Is getting in shape important for my lifestyle?

A: Hey! Round is a shape!

And please take note of the conclusion arrived at by the interviewer/author of this little gem. Chuckle, but please realize that we're dealing here with large doses of satire and facetiousness:

For those of you who watch what you eat, here's the final word on nutrition and health. It's a relief to know the truth after all those conflicting nutritional studies.

1. Japanese eat very little fat and suffer fewer heart attacks than Americans.
2. Mexicans eat a lot of fat and suffer fewer heart attacks than Americans.
3. Chinese drink very little red wine and suffer fewer heart attacks than Americans.
4. Italians drink a lot of red wine and suffer fewer heart attacks than Americans.
5. Germans drink a lot of beers and eat lots of sausages and fats and suffer fewer heart attacks than Americans.

CONCLUSION
EAT AND DRINK WHAT YOU LIKE.
SPEAKING ENGLISH IS APPARENTLY WHAT KILLS YOU!!!

Now let's get serious again.

may be issues for very young children as well as people of our age. And obesity is a major health problem in our society in both childhood and adulthood. But certain medical issues are more prevalent in the Boomer years and in stages beyond.

The good news is that exercise can either modify the potency of some of these undesirable conditions or reduce the likelihood of their appearance in the first place. Among the ways that exercise accomplishes this is by fortifying your *immune system* (see Chapter 1). To make this point, let's consider three illnesses in particular that often present themselves in the

Boomer years and see how each relates to exercise. These three illnesses are osteoporosis, colon cancer, and diabetes.

OSTEOPOROSIS

Your skeletal system serves as a scaffold for your muscles and ligaments. Think of your body's long bones (legs, arms) as levers that muscles move by contracting and relaxing. Exercise strengthens your bones and increases their density. In order to get about safely and efficiently while maintaining a high level of health and fitness, your bony framework must be kept in tip-top condition. When the amount of bone mass (density) of your bones diminishes, they are more susceptible to fracture. Bone density decreases as we advance from early adulthood to old and older adulthood.

A condition that involves thinning and weakening of bones, quite common in older women, is *osteoporosis*. In older women an increased risk of fracture puts the spine, hip, and wrist in particular jeopardy, although osteoporosis is by no means restricted to these anatomical parts, or for that matter, to women. Men and children may also be afflicted, but women, more so.

Although no specific symptoms are associated with osteoporosis, frequent bone breaks are often the telltale sign. Therefore, it's a very good idea to have a bone mineral test known as a *dexascan* (noninvasive and painless—akin to an X-ray) in order to determine your bone mass. Women have smaller bones than men and after menopause hormonal changes cause their bone tissue to lose density more rapidly. Another contributing factor is that in general, both older men and women have poorer balance and vision than younger persons. Balance and vision may not be acutely reduced and may certainly be adequate in the elderly, but they are often not what they were earlier in life. Many older persons are, therefore, more prone to falling. And falls often result in broken bones. (Have another look at Chapter 1 where I talked about falling.)

Another indication of osteoporosis is a reduction in skeletal height. If you notice a loss of more than one inch in skeletal height as you age it might very well be that a series of spinal column fractures has occurred and that you have osteoporosis.

Avoiding Osteoporosis

Diets rich in vitamin D and calcium can help prevent loss of bone mass. So can exercise. Since muscular strength, flexibility, and balance are improved by regular physical activity, the likelihood of taking a spill is reduced. Leg strength, understandably critical in maintaining stability, can deter loss of balance and subsequent falling. Weight-bearing exercises such as walking, jogging, and weight-lifting strengthen the bones, so that if you should fall, the probability of fracture is lessened. High impact exercise should be avoided when your physician diagnoses osteoporosis.

A link has been established between tobacco smoking and low bone density. Fearful of appearing preachy, let me only say that a word to the wise should be sufficient on this account.

COLON CANCER

Exercise—particularly the aerobic kind—stimulates the wave-like movement of the muscles lining the colon known as *peristalsis*, which moves the byproducts of digestion in the large intestine toward the anal opening, through which they are excreted. In this manner, material that your body can't use is disposed of. Your colon is like a waste disposal plant. Digestive residue hanging around the colon too long can become toxic and leak out into your otherwise healthy tissues, thus interfering with their normal and proper function and prompting them to become cancerous. Exercise encourages movement of this debris and hastens it toward its intended natural exit. So reports Dr. Kathleen Wolin and colleagues of the Washington University School of Medicine in St. Louis[1] after careful review of the scientific literature.

Another related benefit of exercise is that it represses the development of other cancer risk factors such as obesity and diabetes. In short, exercise, or at least a physically active lifestyle, can decrease the risk of colon cancer significantly.[2] Considering that colorectal cancer is the second-leading cause of death for both men and women in the United States, there are tremendous health implications for physical activity.

We know that cancer itself and the chemical and radiological treatments prescribed to combat it tend to suppress the immune system. Exercise can countermand this suppression and in fact strengthen immune system function. Some evidence indicates that nausea, commonly reported by breast cancer patients receiving chemotherapy, is relieved following aerobic exercise.[3] Exercise also enables patients undergoing chemotherapy to retain or even increase their energy levels, muscular strength, and endurance, which often wane during therapy, thus enhancing their functional capacities.

You can legitimately conclude that exercise, especially aerobic exercise, plays significant roles in cancer prevention as well as management of the disease itself once it has been diagnosed. Bottom line: a sedentary lifestyle (and according to Cedric Bryant, Chief Science Officer of the American Council of Exercise, as much as 50% of the entire North American population is sedentary) significantly increases the risk of cancer, especially breast cancer. This is what Dr. Anne McTiernan, Director of the Fred Hutchinson Cancer Research Center's prevention Center in Seattle, Washington, tells us.

My message is simple: Keep moving to reduce the probability of bumping into cancer! Dr. Steven Blair, noted expert on exercise and health, maintains that the percent of inactive American adults is somewhere between 25 and 35 (sedentary jobs, no regular physical activity program, and in general, inactive around the house or yard). Speaking at the American Psychological Association's 117th Annual Convention in 2009, Dr. Blair indicted the sedentary lifestyle of American adults as the biggest public health problem of the 21st century. As the lyrics to a song popularized not too long ago in the animated film, *Madagascar*, you've got to "move it, move it." So dive into the wellspring of available physical activity options. Surface with one that seems right for you—and DO IT!

DIABETES

Exercise is a potent weapon to incorporate into your lifestyle if you are diabetic. It can be of significant benefit. Here's why.

Glucose, or blood sugar is required for proper functioning of all your body's cells. A hormone produced in your pancreas, known as *insulin*, is needed to transport blood glucose to the body's cells. If there is inadequate production or supply of insulin, the condition of *insulin-dependent diabetes mellitus* (also known as *Type 1)* exists. If you are unable to produce adequate amounts of insulin you must receive it through injection. *Type 2* or *noninsulin-dependent diabetes mellitus* involves adequate production and supply of insulin, but for some reason the hormone is ineffective in transporting glucose to the body's cells. In other words, insulin does not do its assigned job. Eighty to ninety percent of all diabetics have the Type 2 kind, which involves too much sugar in the blood. This is a serious problem in that the body reacts in very negative and potentially harmful ways in the face of glucose imbalance.

Physical activity improves your ability to utilize insulin and lowers your blood glucose levels since your muscles require relatively more fuel during exercise. You'll use more glucose when exercising. In addition, your body fat is likely to be reduced over a period of time as your metabolism increases and you burn additional calories. Since exercise has an insulin-like effect on the body and tends to lower blood sugar values, it's important to monitor your sugar level before, during, and after exercise if you are diabetic. It is also possible that your glucose level may be at dangerously low levels and that exercise can lower it even more. The term *hypoglycemia* refers to blood sugar levels that are too low. Some signs of hypoglycemia during exercise are excessive sweating, confusion, changes in heartbeat, increased anxiety, and hunger.

If you are diabetic and the above symptoms occur, stop exercising immediately. In advanced cases of diabetes, damage to nerves in the extremities may have occurred and sensitivity in the feet and toes may be reduced. If you are an exercising diabetic you may therefore not be aware of injury, which may lead to serious complications. Wear comfortable and proper shoes when participating in exercise. Follow all the cautions and advice that I've been offering throughout this book as you engage in vigorous physical activity. If you have blood pressure, blood vessel, or eye problems (as many diabetics do), stay away from heavy weight training. We'll have much more to say about injury in Chapters 5 and 6.

FROM ME TO YOU—APOLOGIA

Exercise is not the miraculous snake oil that will prevent or cure all illness or malaise—of course not. Furthermore, I assure you that I do not expect you to adopt my degree of enthusiasm for physical activity. It would be unfair, unwise, and inappropriate for me to have such an aspiration. I know this. On the other hand, don't conveniently adopt an exercise-deprived lifestyle simply because others seem to be okay without it. We all know individuals who have defied expert nutritional advice and recommendations for healthy living and yet have lived surprisingly extended lives. The implication here is that they never exercised regularly—never needed to—because they are genetically endowed. In other words, it's all about genes.

Conventional wisdom indeed suggests that these persons have inherited exceptional physiological protectors that somehow advantage them. But don't wager that you are similarly benefited even if these unusual people are family members. Don't use them as models. Most of us also know individuals who have survived incredible assaults upon their bodies—war, auto accidents, and serious physical trauma—and their very survival is in defiance of their doctor's considered prognosis. They endure and do nicely. My advice is to avoid making lifestyle decisions based upon what you've observed in these exceptional people.

I'm not prophesying doom. Not at all. I'm asking you to incorporate exercise into your life on a regular basis simply because it's an excellent investment. It not only has the capacity to elevate your present quality of life, health, and wellness, but it can strengthen your organic readiness to confront illness or compromised health in the future. It offers no guarantee for immortality or disease-free living. But it can be your inexpensive ticket to a fun-filled, healthy existence.

Some form of exercise is readily available to everyone and because you have no way of knowing what your genetic profile looks like and what it portends, undertake programmatic exercise as insurance against future organic/structural breakdowns. Don't delude yourself into believing that you'll probably enjoy the same benefits as the guy who ate, drank, and smoked excessively and lived to be one hundred while thumbing his nose at exercise zealots like me. Don't use these exceptional and fortunate persons as a reason for avoiding regular exercise.

And excuse me if I come across as being too fervent in my advocacy. But I read the scientific studies. I've done my own research, guided the research of others, read the books, and done this for decades. I want my enthusiasm for regular physical activity to be contagious yet rational.

Something else for you to chew on: In two fairly recent studies conducted by the U.S. Department of Energy's Lawrence Berkley National Laboratory, one eye-popping (pun intended) conclusion was that vigorous cardiovascular (aerobic) exercise may be an excellent way to ward off *cataracts* and age-related *macular degenerative disease*. I suspect that many of you are well informed about both of these afflictions.

☞ WHAT YOU'VE LEARNED IN THIS CHAPTER

Wellness and health are not the same. You can be unhealthy but well, or unwell and quite healthy. A high degree of wellness means that the major parts of your life (social, mental, emotional, physical, and spiritual) are satisfactorily attended to and in balance. Even if confronted with a diagnosis of terminal cancer you can be very well if you have supportive friends and relatives (social), if your emotions are in check (emotional), if you are receiving excellent medical care and medication that controls your pain and discomfort (physical), if you have a thorough understanding of the limitations and consequences imposed by your illness (mental), and if you have religious beliefs and faith that provide comfort and hope (spiritual).

The chapter also explained the role of exercise in achieving and sustaining high levels of both health and wellness. It clarified how physical activity can help prevent and manage some illnesses common to the over-60 crowd, notably osteoporosis, colon cancer, and diabetes. Although not a cure-all for these maladies, exercise can play a significant role in their prevention and alleviation.

FOOD FOR THOUGHT	
1	Assess the degree of balance among the major dimensions of your life. Take a look at your social component. Are your relationships with relatives solid? Do you have intimate friendships that allow for exchange of confidences? What is your self-view with regard to emotionality? Do you fly off the handle easily? Are you frequently anxious? And are your coping mechanisms for dealing with anxiety adequate?
2	Have you undergone a thorough medical examination during the past year? Do you understand all aspects of your physician's diagnoses and results of various medical tests that you've had? Is the information provided by your physician acceptable to you? Do you believe that a second opinion is necessary?
3	What is your reaction to the notion that exercise has illness prevention capabilities?

Endnotes

1. Wolin, K., Yan, Y., Colditz, G.A., & Lee, I-M. (2009).
2. 2006.
3. 2008.

Chapter 3

EATING RIGHT AND FEELING GOOD: NUTRITIONAL CONSIDERATIONS

Rachel wants to lose weight. With the passing years she has gradually accumulated unwanted fat around the hips and thighs. She is bothered by this and is conscious of her husband's notice of her change in body shape. Although he says nothing, she suspects that it bothers him as well. She has cut down on carbohydrates and sweets but is unable to drop the excessive poundage. Rachel is borderline diabetic and her physician has encouraged her to lose 20–35 pounds. He tells her that if this doesn't happen soon, two outcomes are likely: 1) she'll continue to put on more weight, and 2) her diabetic tendency will become full blown. Rachel is 67 and gets no exercise whatsoever.

According to Greek mythology Narcissus, an unusually handsome young man, was curiously indifferent to the advances and adoration offered by the bevies of gorgeous maidens who fervently pursued him. His unseemly disinterest was noted by the gods who consequently inflicted upon him a rather

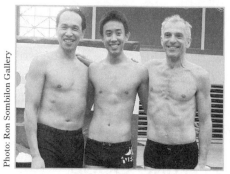

How others see you and
how you see yourself
can have an enormous
impact on your
psychology.

severe punishment. He was made to fall in love with his own reflection in a mountain pool. And because he was unable to possess this image, his unrequited love caused him to pine away. He eventually expired and turned into a flower. Quite a story— but the point is, your physical appearance and your assumptions about how others see you, as well as the view you hold about yourself, have enormous impact upon your psychology.

I've made this point in other chapters; however, it merits reemphasis. Although I've arbitrarily used the case of Rachel in the scenario to open this chapter, be assured that I could have just as easily presented a hypothetical male counterpart. Perhaps more so than in other parts of the world, in Western society both women and men look critically at their body shapes. Our cultural directives prompt this. Mirrors abound in the places and rooms we habituate, and we are not loathe to glance at our image in passing. When assessment results in dissatisfaction, a desire to change often follows.

In large measure your physical appearance is determined by hereditary factors. Genes inherited from forbearers establish your skeletal framework, and you have nothing to say about their presence or impact. There's little you can do, short of drastic surgery, to alter their influence. But with effort you can modify some of the physical attributes accounted for by genes.

On the one hand, the dimensions of your shoulders—whether they slope a bit or are squared, are not discretionary—they are genetically determined. But with weight training and other forms of exercise, you can influence the amount of muscle mass covering the shoulder area and the manner in which your arms move in and around the shoulder joint. On the other hand, if the way in which your hair sits on your head displeases you, curling, coloring, or straightening it in order to conform to the latest fashion is indeed an option. You can also regulate your body weight through diet and exercise. And this is precisely the major focus of this chapter. In this chapter I'll discuss various aspects of diet, nutrition, body weight, and fat storage and depletion—all in relation to exercise, and of course, with particular application to the over-60 crowd.

Countless diet and nutrition books are on the market, many of which are well written and contain accurate and helpful information. I recommend that you have a look at one or two of them. They are available in abundance at your local bookstores. Here I want to provide but a brief, and admittedly, somewhat superficial overview of some of the salient aspects of these topics because dietary and nutritional issues are so very clearly integral to health, well-being, and exercise.

By way of introducing the discussion, let me indicate a difference between the terms *nutrition* and *diet*. Both, of course, refer to ingestion of food, but the important difference is that nutrition concerns the science or study of foodstuff with major attention devoted to biochemical and physiological factors. In contrast, words such as *diet* or *dietary* apply when concern is focused upon what is contained in the meals you eat. Nutritionists study food ingredients such as fats, minerals, proteins, and carbohydrates, while dieticians are concerned with eating patterns and menus. At times the missions of these two areas overlap.

THE SELF-VIEW: BODY IMAGE

We all hold a particular view of our physical selves, namely the *body image*. Narcissus' perspective was one of self-adoration. For this he paid dearly. Your body image is but one of numerous self-views, among them being views of your social, intellectual, and emotional selves. Basically defined as the mental picture you have of your physicality, body image has been determined in study after study to be a foundational element of your psychology.

Strong and clear connections exist between the image you have of your body and its parts, and evaluations you make about many other dimensions of yourself. A link between body image and the manner in which you deport yourself—how you perform daily interactions with others in your social environment—has also been established. When you believe that your body is functioning well, when you like how you move or what you see in the mirror, your overall assessment of yourself (*self-concept*) is enhanced and strengthened. Your spirits are elevated; you feel good. When you move with precision and aplomb, or if you perform in some physical way with courage and efficiency, your body image is strengthened. And reciprocally, when your body image is bolstered, you tend to perform well.

Findings in a recently published study by French scientists[1] are apropos of what we're talking about here. The study measured 8,600 women over the age of 60 and found that they routinely overestimated their height by an inch. As we age we lose height because discs between the vertebrae in the spine compress. But the women in this study viewed themselves as being taller than they really were.

Very similar findings were reported for American men and women in an older study.[2] In this research the error in self-reported body weight was found to be related to age in women. The older the woman, the greater the discrepancy. Why? Perhaps an effort to protect or enhance the body image is accountable. Or maybe cultural imperatives dictated this error (or deception). We can't be sure.

Another study[3] employed more than 7,000 men and 8,000 women of various ages starting at age 20. Among the findings: both men and women over 70 overestimated their height (believed that they were taller than they actually were) and underestimated their body weight. Younger participants in the study did not demonstrate errors in estimation as large as the older subjects. Bottom line of all three studies: Self reported heights and weights are much more accurate in younger adults than in men and women more than 60 years of age. This suggests that the latter are in danger of being misclassified when standard weight tables are used for medical purposes and body weights are solicited from the patients themselves. They may not be reporting accurate weights.

Physical appearance is an important exercise incentive for men and women of all ages because through exercise the body's shape can be somewhat redesigned. When and if you succeed in this reshaping, your interactions with others tend to become more confident and pleasurable. True, exercise will not enable you to alter your skeletal height, since bone growth usually stops in the late teens, but as noted a few paragraphs previously, body weight and muscular development may certainly be modified. In short, you feel good about your body when you believe it looks and functions well. And this good feeling may easily generalize to other parts of your self-concept. One way to alter your physical appearance, and thus the image you hold of it, is by manipulating the amount of body fat stored beneath your skin.

FAT STORAGE AND FAT METABOLISM

To be healthy and well, you need body fat. (We talked about this need in Chapter 1.) A certain amount of fat is good, so don't completely disparage its presence. Fat is important in that it protects the internal organs, helps with body temperature regulation (insulation), and provides shape to your physique. But too much stored body fat is problematic—not just from the aesthetic point of view, which is culturally influenced, but from the health standpoint. The more body fat you collect and keep, the more you weigh. In a nutshell, the more you weigh, the greater the load on your cardiorespiratory mechanisms. In other words, your heart and lungs must work harder to provide nourishment (blood and oxygen) to all of your body tissues.

Consider the following analogy: When you load up your automobile with furniture lashed to the roof, when the trunk is full and the rear seat is packed with boxes and luggage, your engine strains as it functions. When proceeding uphill, the engine works even harder.

Such is the case with your heart and its mandate to distribute blood and its essential elements throughout the body. If the amount of fat you carry is excessive to the extent that you are *obese* (at least one-third over your ideal body weight), then your heart is obliged to labor under an unfair and dangerous load. The respiratory system must work harder in order to bring in more air and get rid of waste gas. When increased demands during exercise are put upon your cardiorespiratory mechanisms, they are additionally taxed. Muscles require more oxygen and nutriment during exercise and more heat is produced, which increases sweating. Overweight definitely carries physical liabilities and imposes significant burdens in all your organs and physiological systems.

Whereas exercise done regularly over the long term can reduce stored body fat, the irony is that the heart and circulatory system must function at very high and sometimes dangerous levels during a bout of exercise. Therein lies the rub. If you are very overweight, exercise may not be the preferred method for body fat reduction—at least in the beginning.

This is not to disparage physical activity as a weight regulation strategy. Certainly not, because a very beneficial cumulative effect of exercise is possible whereby small and relatively light doses of exercise "collected" over time may very significantly enhance your fitness level and reduce body weight. You need not burn body fat in one fell swoop. It can be done gradually. But you cannot claim a reasonably high degree of physical fitness and be over-fat.

Mind you, I'm only speaking of excess amounts of stored body fat, not necessarily gross body weight. An Olympic heavyweight wrestler or boxer, or professional football player may weigh more than one third over his ideal body weight, but his overweight may very well not be due to fat storage. Muscle mass may be the relevant factor. It would be best to first lose some body weight, thereby reducing onerous loads on the circulatory and respiratory systems, and then begin an appropriately designed exercise regimen.

I'll have more to say about depletion of unwanted body fat through diet and exercise in the paragraphs and pages that follow. At any rate, consultation with a physician in order to determine you are ready for rigorous exercise is a preferred first step in any weight reduction program involving exercise. This is important in order to determine the extent to which rigorous exercise is appropriate.

FAT AND CULTURE

Before I delve into the mechanisms underlying fat storage, let me return very briefly to a comment I offered previously about culture having an impact upon the way a society views people with fat storage tendencies. Some cultures are particularly severe in their condemnation of those who carry considerable amounts of body fat. Others actually condone and reinforce it. In 17th and 18th century Europe, men with large protruding bellies and folds beneath their chin were considered to be prosperous and attractive; poor men struggled to put food on the table and were scrawny. For years many South Pacific nations evaluated men to be very virile and macho who our contemporary culture would deem obese. Cultural anthropologists tell us that in Polynesian societies perhaps as recently as 100 years ago, exceedingly heavy women were also seen as attractive and thin ones, uncomely. If you have the opportunity, take a look at photos or portraits of Hawaiian queens of yesteryear and notice their abundance of flesh. It seems that regal status was typically associated with corpulence. Not so in present Western society where thin has been in for quite some time and a lean prototype is promoted for physical attractiveness. Fashion magazines today clearly favor a comparatively svelte look, and models portrayed as handsome or attractive are svelte and spare.

HOW AND WHERE IS FAT STORED?

Fat cells are present in your blood and in many of your internal organs, such as the liver. However, our concern here is with fatty tissue located under your skin and surrounding your internal organs. The former you can feel and be aware of. Your mirror and belt provide feedback. If you starved yourself, you would ultimately relinquish blood and liver fat, but this of course is not what I'm advocating. No one is encouraging you to starve, but you should understand that middle age as well as

Boomer status and beyond are associated with increasingly greater storage of body fat. As we age we tend to store more fat.

Your daily caloric requirement varies according to your gender, age, weight, and lifestyle. Let's arbitrarily say your need is somewhere around 2,500 calories per day (younger persons require more calories, and most males require more than females). If your daily intake dips below 600 you are technically starving. Again, I'm not promoting starvation. I'm just defining the term.

When someone expresses a wish to lose weight through diet and exercise, in effect he or she is contemplating one or two strategies: 1) using up fat stored under the skin by reducing caloric intake and 2) increasing caloric requirements by ratcheting up physical activity. A minimal number of calories are necessary to fuel basic metabolic requirements. The efforts of body organs and systems require fuel, namely calories. These calories—understood by scientists to be units of heat—are introduced via the foods you eat. Foods vary in their caloric content. A dish of ice cream has many, celery relatively few. The more calories you bring in beyond what your metabolism requires, the more this energy is stored in the form of body fat.

A brief overview of a few concepts and terms should enable you to better understand how and where body fat is stored. Then you'll be positioned to relate this knowledge to exercise.

Adipose tissues are the highly specialized safety deposit boxes located under the skin where fat cells congregate. Some places in your body have more of this tissue than others, and some persons have relatively greater amounts of this kind of tissue than others (heredity). Therefore, the tendency to store fat varies among us, as do the likely places for its storage. All of us have a predetermined number of deflated fat cells that reside in adipose tissue. They are waiting to be filled. The number of fat cells is determined very early in life and is stabilized during childhood. When you bring in more calories than you need, these cells fill, and fat is stored. Exercise can reduce the size of these fat cells.[4]

Many decades of living have revealed your very particular locations for fat deposition—for instance, the hips, neck, face, or chest. You know where your stored fat reveals itself. Unfortunately, you have no choice in the matter of where your adipose tissue is situated. Fat will be stored where adipose tissue and empty fat cells exist and their amount and location is genetically determined. You entered this world with designated amounts and locations of adipose tissue.

When your body yields its fat, it does so in accordance with an enigmatic and often frustrating order of priority. Though you can come to know which areas of your body are most likely to relinquish fat first or last, you can't influence the order in which it occurs. Although you need some measure of body fat, be aware that like all other tissues, adipose must be nourished. This means that during physical activity (or even at rest), it too needs servicing and nourishment, thereby further burdening the circulatory and respiratory systems.

Another concept that should enable you to better understand fat storage is known as *thermodynamic theory*, which I briefly discussed in Chapter 1. Its explanation of how fat is deposited and how body weight is lost or gained is based upon the notion of energy–in/energy–out. Here's a simple version: The more calories you consume in excess of what you need, the more fat you'll store. The more calories you use in excess of what your body requires, the more fat you'll give up and the more weight you'll lose.

The term *thermo* derives from the Greek (therme) and refers to heat, which brings us back to the word calorie, essentially a unit of heat or energy. When the food you eat is oxidized or burned, heat is given off. Therefore, one popular approach to understanding weight gain and loss is through the idea of heat or energy balance, or *thermodynamics*.

Of course, there are additional considerations that compound this basic but attractive explanation. Some people have unusual metabolic requirements and fat-storing mechanisms that undermine the simplicity of the thermodynamics approach. Perhaps you know of people whose *basal metabolic function* (the rate of cellular activity at rest) is so low that they require very little food and few calories. This being the case, they satisfy their caloric need very easily and convert a good deal of what they eat into stored body fat. Put in terms of a bank savings account, these individuals are very parsimonious and save fat more efficiently than others who "spend" (or utilize or burn it) more readily.

Although elderly status brings with it many delightful benefits, it also conveys a tendency toward increased body fat storage. You require fewer daily calories since your metabolic rate has lowered somewhat. Exercise is one readily available way to countermand such tendencies. The elusive fountain of youth, if it actually exists, may very well be found in the food you eat and the amount you eat.

Quite a few published studies conclude that caloric restriction in combination with exercise increases longevity in rodents. These findings although interesting, have not yet been sufficiently supported in studies using humans. I've talked about mouse and rat studies previously and cautioned about the appropriateness of assuming the transferability of rodent studies to the human condition. What's good for the goose may very well be good for the gander, but in this case, what's good for the mouse may not necessarily be good for us.

EATING DISORDERS

Unusual eating patterns that have bearing upon fat storage or depletion are referred to with the term *eating disorders*. Among the most well known of these are *anorexia nervosa* and *bulimia*. Both bring to mind problematical psychological issues and both require professional intervention by trained and qualified mental health professionals. I discuss these two unfortunate conditions in case some persons you know (e.g., grandchildren, nephews, nieces) demonstrate characteristics or symptoms that bring them to mind.

The first condition, *anorexia*, is characterized by intentional, acute deprivation of caloric iintake. Affected individuals starve themselves because they are under the distinct but absolutely fallacious impression that they are overweight. Despite attempts by caring relatives and friends to convince them otherwise, anorectics hold grossly inaccurate perceptions of their body image and are pathologically fearful of being overweight.

If anything, they are significantly underweight, but are unable to see their bodies as such.

By depriving themselves of their most basic caloric needs, people with anorexia inflict upon themselves serious physiological damage that may eventually culminate in death. They starve themselves and force their internal organs to release protein (I'll comment upon this food component a little later). The essential building blocks of your vital organs are proteins. Organs that sacrifice a portion of their supply of this foodstuff compromise their structural integrity and seriously weaken their functions. When numerous organs are damaged in this way, critical body chemistry is dramatically and detrimentally altered. The result can be extremely serious—death by starvation.

One additional factor makes a discussion of anorexia pertinent here. Anorexia is often accompanied by frequent and abusive exercise. Too much exercise can cause great harm, and people with anorexia are often guilty of overexercising. Their exercise regimens are obsessively intense, compulsive, and over the top. In such cases it's biologically traumatic and injurious. They exaggerate the narrative delivered in a catchy tune embedded in the wonderful animated film I referred to previously, called *Madagascar*: "I like to move it, move it, move it." They move it so excessively that their health, well-being, and very life are threatened.

Another eating disorder, *bulimia*, involves purging (use of laxatives or self-induced vomiting) following binge eating. Bulimics tend to be chubby and usually have a superfluous amount of stored body fat, but they are not always dramatically overweight or obese. Bulimics gorge and then very soon, surreptitiously, get rid of what they've consumed.

Although anorexia and bulimia may afflict persons of all ages, young people are most commonly affected. Perhaps this is because young people are just developing their body image, whereas you and I probably long ago resolved such matters. The likelihood of your falling prey to these two conditions at your age is remote (but possible). This is not the case with your young relatives, neighbors, and acquaintances.

My parting comment on this topic is cautionary. Both of

these eating disorders are very serious and absolutely require professional attention because they may be linked to a psychological or codependent disorder. The best thing you can do to assist persons whom you suspect of being in the grip of these afflictions is to see to it that they are directed to competent mental health professionals. Topic closed.

APPETITE VERSUS HUNGER

While discussing dietary and nutritional matters vis-à-vis exercise, health, and wellness, two relevant and distinct terms require clarification. They should not be used interchangeably.

Appetite is psychological and refers to the desire to seek and eat food. This desire may be encouraged by any number of environmental stimulants: a photo of food, people around you eating, or an association of food with time of day or physical location. Your stomach may actually be quite full, yet your appetite keen. Appetite is not necessarily curbed by recent eating or by how much you've just eaten. When your appetite is edgy and your interest in food activated, you tend to eat, and eat a lot. The result is high caloric intake, and if your caloric expenditure is minimal (little exercise or physical activity), increased fat storage is the consequence (thermodynamics).

Hunger, on the other hand, is physiological and detectible when your digestive system is virtually empty of food and your body cells have been deprived of nourishment. Sensory nerve endings positioned in various areas of the digestive system send messages indicating the biological need for food to your brain, which registers sensations of discomfort. You become aware of your hunger.

Although perception (interpretation of sensations) is involved in hunger, psychological processes are not paramount. It's essentially a biological issue. When you are hungry, your body is shouting, "Send down food! Your cells and tissues are calorie deprived!" In contrast, when appetite is stimulated, your belly's fullness or emptiness is irrelevant. You may be attracted to food, or at least certain kinds of food, even though you have recently eaten well.

Under normal circumstances, as you age, you require fewer calories and this reduced need should be reflected in the amount of food you eat. How many calories do you require? The answer depends on a number of factors: your gender, the amount of physical activity you do daily, your body weight, and genetic determinants. A rough estimate of the daily caloric requirement for maintaining your current body weight would be approximately 1,800 if you are an active female Boomer. If you are male the number would be about 2,400.

Above and beyond the number of calories required to fuel daily activity, about 3,500 calories account for one pound of stored body fat. As soon as you hit this number, beyond your daily metabolic need, you'll put on a pound of fat—somewhere. But in order to lose a pound of fat your caloric intake must be reduced by approximately 3,300 calories. Adding this pound requires a little energy which is not required to lose it. Putting on pounds during aging has become so common in our society that it seems to be a natural course of events. This creeping weight gain is neither desirable nor unavoidable; older people should be no fatter than younger people.

ARE YOU TOO FAT?

Proper weight is not only determined by checking your bathroom scale. Body mass index (BMI) is a widely used metric for ascertaining overweight and obesity and is fairly easy to calculate. What it provides is a rough estimation of your stored body fat. Here's the formula:

The product of 'weight in pounds' × '703' (a) divided by the product of 'height in inches' × 'height in inches' (b) = 'bmi' (c) [a / b = c].

If your BMI is below 18.5 you are underweight; 18.5–24.9 is the normal range; 25–29.9 means that you are overweight; 30+ would designate you as obese.

But BMI is far from perfect as a measure of the body's fat content because it may permit inaccurate classification of nonobesity. The system provides for an approximation of stored fat based only on overall body weight and skeletal height. It really only makes assumptions about the weight of your muscle tissue.

When results of the BMI calculations are compared with those generated by more costly and time-consuming assessment procedures that zero in on fat storage alone, the BMI data don't compare favorably. Examples of these superior techniques are underwater weighing and skin-fold measurement. Too many people assessed by BMI are not identified as obese. Also, racial differences, especially in women, tend to bear upon the calculation. The same is probably true with regard to men, but I've yet to find support for this in the scientific literature.

And don't forget that as we advance into old age we tend to shrink a bit. Therefore, as we become more and more elderly the BMI would be higher (the skeletal height variable becomes smaller) even if body fat doesn't increase. Although popularly employed today, I suggest that if you are really interested in how much of your total body weight comprises fat, you would be best served by using other tools.[5]

To simply maintain proper and healthful body weight, if you are over 60, the party line dictates that you should eat fewer calories. Muscle mass and bone density decrease during this period of life and therefore even though the scale may reveal no change in overall body weight, the likelihood of an increase in stored fat is high. Ideally, your weight need not, and should not, increase as you get older. You were probably at an ideal body weight during your 20s and after age 60 you should strive to maintain this level.

Foodstuffs: Basic Ingredients of What You Eat

Food is something you naturally dwell upon throughout the day. If you are like me, you plan eating times and think about where and when and perhaps with whom you'd like to eat. Your stomach is practically empty five to seven hours after eating and intricate physiological interactions signal the brain that it's time to do it again. Since you have been conditioned to anticipate this cycle, predicting when you will be hungry is not difficult and you are able to make luncheon and dinner appointments days and even weeks in advance.

All food consists of *nutrients* upon which life depends. The fuel that energizes cellular activity comes mostly from what you eat. Chemists and nutritionists have special words for food components and talk about fats, proteins, carbohydrates, vitamins, and minerals, whereas most of us use words like *steak*, *tomato*,

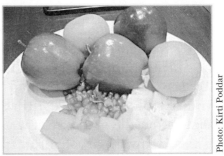

Photo: Kirti Poddar

All food consists of nutrients upon which life depends. What kind of nutrients are in your food?

bread, and *apple*. Food components differ from one another in their chemical construction and are present in different foods in varying degrees. Potato has more carbohydrate than carrot, and carrot more vitamin A than potato.

For most of us it is not much of a challenge to satisfy daily carbohydrate, fat, protein, vitamin, mineral, and water requirements. Our typical diet enables this, although malnutrition is certainly not unknown in many contemporary societies. A few comments about each of these foodstuffs are now in order—nothing complicated or highly detailed, just some information that should make it easier to understand your fundamental nutritional and dietary needs. Upon beginning an exercise program it's necessary to be in touch with basic nutritional requirements and concept. I begin with water because it is the most critical component of your diet. Without it you don't just gradually starve to death in a few weeks—you die in very short order (a few days).

WATER

Water has zero calories. But don't dare minimize its dietary importance. A good 70% of what's in each and every one of your body cells is water. Most of your blood is nothing more than water. You absolutely need water.

Your age and the amount of muscle and fat tissue you have determine the amount of water you require. Muscle holds more water than fat. Unless it is artificially fortified, water contains no nutrients, but it can nonetheless add weight to your body. Try this: Stand on a bathroom scale, weigh yourself, and while you're still on the scale, drink a glass of water. You'll notice that the needle moves; you weigh more.

A diet low in carbohydrate (pastry, bread, pasta, etc.) will result in rapid water loss because carbohydrates bond with water. Now you understand why some of the popular weight loss regimens on the market claim dramatic weight loss results during the first 10 days. Most of what is lost is water weight that is almost immediately restored when a few glasses of water are drunk.

You can survive for weeks with food but only a few days without water. But can you take in too much of it? There have been a few cases in which people overhydrate and end up in trouble (*hyponatremia*) and die—mostly athletes and overzealous jocks. Not to worry. This condition is rare and if you bring in more than you need, you'll just urinate more and unload it. On average for all ages, adult women need about 8 glasses of water per day—men, about 12. So goes the conventional wisdom. But take into consideration that you drink tea, coffee (when black it contains virtually no calories), and soda. The fruits and vegetables you eat also contain substantial amounts of water. Although about 80% of your requirement comes from drinking water, as long as your intake somehow includes the equivalent of 8 or 12 glasses, you'll be okay.

When the water level in your body is too low, the sensation of thirst tells you so. A special group of nerve cells in the brain's hypothalamus is sensitive to the body's water supply and sends thirst signals to other brain centers, so you develop an awareness of what's going on.

Physical activity increases water loss and therefore elevates your need. If you are exercising, drink more water. Your body cells need to be hydrated before and, if possible, during physical activity. Carry bottled water with you when out for a walk or when working in the yard, but only for convenience sake, not because bottled water is in any way superior to what runs from your tap. Your local board of health regulates the purity and contents of the community's supply and thus guarantees a healthy and usually inexpensive product. You need increased amounts of water during rigorous physical activity to satisfy various and complex biochemical reactions in your muscle tissue. You also require water for body temperature regulation and to facilitate circulatory function. Adequate amounts of water are also required for digestion of food, as well as joint lubrication and healthy skin.

CARBOHYDRATES

Carbohydrates are a very important source of energy for muscular activity. Most foods contain carbohydrates that your body eventually converts to simple sugars. An example of simple sugar would be the white granular material found in a jar on the local diner's lunch counter—the stuff you spoon into your tea or coffee cup. But simple sugars are also found in foods that have high nutritional value such as milk, fruit, pasta, and rice. Milk and fruit are better sources of carbohydrates than simple sugar because they also provide other important ingredients.

Simple sugars make their way into your blood stream quickly but provide only a fleeting energy boost, and you are therefore likely to be hungry again soon. You probably consume more carbohydrate than protein in your daily diet because foods high in carbohydrates are typically cheap and those rich in protein comparatively expensive. Bread products, potato, and rice are examples of the former, and beef, fish, poultry and eggs, of the latter. Foods referred to as *staples* are high in carbohydrates and are basic dietary components throughout the world (once again, rice, pasta, bread, etc.).

The cell walls of cereal grain seeds, vegetable leaves, and stems are high in a fibrous form of carbohydrate and referred to with the term *fiber*. Fiber stimulates proper digestive function. It is not broken down by your body's natural chemicals and remains in the lower intestine and retains water that is helpful in bowel movement. Most foods obtained from animal sources contain little or no carbohydrate.

FAT

Animals and vegetables are common sources of dietary fat. Fats derived from plant sources are said to be *unsaturated* and are usually liquid. Animal sources provide *saturated* fat and tend to be hard. Liver, red meats, egg yolk, and butter are examples of foods high in *cholesterol*, a soft waxy material which has been linked to cardiovascular disease. Cholesterol derives its name from Greek *chole*, meaning *bile* and *steros*, meaning *solid*. It is not found in plants. However, the amount in your blood is not due exclusively to dietary factors. Your body itself manufactures a substantial amount of it.

What makes cholesterol a relevant topic for discussion here is its connection to exercise, fitness, and wellness. Cholesterol may be deposited in the walls of the coronary arteries and hardens into plaques. (Recall the analogy with the clogged garden hose offered in Chapter 1.) Eventually, these plaques result in a narrowing of the blood vessel's diameter, thus making arteries hard (*arteriosclerosis*) and reducing their flexibility. This results in a reduced flow of blood and consequently a reduced amount of oxygen supply to the heart muscle (we also talked about this in Chapter 1). But exercise, aerobic exercise in particular, done regularly over extended periods of time, has the capacity to significantly reduce the amount of cholesterol in your blood (as well as the fat stored beneath the skin). Saturated fats in the diet tend to raise blood cholesterol levels, so it's not just dietary cholesterol that is the problem.

PROTEIN

This foodstuff usually comes from natural dietary animal sources (meat, milk, and eggs, and sometimes plants such as nuts and seeds). After protein is digested, its elements, known as *amino acids*, become building blocks of your cells and tissues. In brief, when you devour a hamburger you are eating the ground tissue (in better quality hamburger meat it's usually muscle tissue) of an animal. The molecules in the protein you've eaten are shuffled, reorganized, and used to fortify or create new muscle tissue or repair damaged organs in your body.

Protein is an essential ingredient in your diet and if deprived of it your body will resort to breaking down its own tissue in an effort to locate a new supply. All of your cell building and regeneration requires protein, and your body is desperate to have it. Hemoglobin, the part of your red blood cells responsible for distributing molecules of oxygen to all body tissues, requires protein, as do all your muscles. Enzymes and neurotransmitters (message carriers) are made of protein as well. Your need for protein increases as you advance chronologically from childhood, but levels off at adulthood. By the time you hit 60, your requirement for this food element is not nearly as great as it was when you were a teenager. Nonetheless, you still require protein in substantial quantities, particularly if you undertake an exercise regimen.

Nine essential amino acids are needed in the protein you eat. Protein that contains all nine are said to be *complete*. Because your body can't manufacture amino acids, they must come from what you eat. Animal sources such as meat and milk provide complete protein, but most vegetable foods are incomplete because they lack one or more of the essential amino acids. So if you are a vegetarian, be careful to load up on vegetables that are reputed to have the amino acids not found in other foods you eat. Be sure to include plenty of legumes (dried beans, peas, and lentils) in your diet.

VITAMINS

There's always much interest in vitamins and vitamin supplements, and I want to be sure you have some basic information about their service to you, with particular emphasis upon their connection to exercise. Advertisements that push these food components in both the print and electronic media are unrelenting. Here's what you need to know.

Dietary vitamins play an important role in maintaining overall good health and tissue growth. Just because you're no longer a child doesn't mean that you are not undergoing continual tissue growth and restructuring. It is this damage/repair routine that eventually generates improved muscle strength and

endurance. Vigorous physical activity that employs large skeletal muscles involves this cycle of cellular damage and repair.
This is why regular exercise should be interspersed with periodic rest intervals in both short- and long-term bases.

Among other things, vitamins fulfill important roles in the regeneration of damaged tissues and the healing processes. But
you actually need only small amounts of these natural food ingredients. They are important because they play a role in the
formulation of enzymes that in turn are necessary for the regulation of your metabolic processes (the functioning of all the little cells in your body). Much greater quantities of carbohydrates
and fats are required because these food elements produce energy; vitamins don't provide fuel for your body. If you are active
and involved in regular exercise, fats and carbohydrates are
needed in substantial amounts. Not so with vitamins.

Vitamins D, E, A, K, folic acid, vitamins B-1, B-2, B-3, B-5,
B-6, and B-12 are examples of *essential* or absolutely necessary
dietary vitamins. A well-balanced diet will provide satisfactory
amounts of these necessities, many of which act in combination
to protect against disease and maintain good health. If your diet
is inadequate or improper, deficiency diseases associated with
specific vitamins are the result. For instance, vitamin D deficiency causes problems with the skeletal system; vitamin E deficiency causes nerve damage; vitamin A deficiency is associated with night vision difficulty; and vitamin B-6 deficiency is
linked to metabolic problems and often with central nervous
system malfunction. Vitamin C is needed for healthy gums and
teeth and the healing of tissue wounds.

Synthetic supplementary vitamins are readily available in local pharmacy or supermarket and can be acquired and used
easily, but only when medical personnel have properly identified a deficiency. You waste your money when you arbitrarily
supplement your diet via self-medication. Such preemptive attempts should be avoided if you have no reason to suspect that
you are vitamin deficient. In fact, the amount of vitamins you
actually need is so low that excessive amounts will be flushed
out of your body by the kidneys. You'll just be urinating away
the unneeded extra stuff. Eating large quantities of vitamins

will not improve your health or promote extraordinary physical feats. You'll not do exercises better if you load up on vitamins.

You would do well to take note of some vitamin-related conditions because they are not uncommon in the elderly. *Pernicious anemia* is an example. It tends to occur in middle or old age more often than in youth. It is associated with damage to the nervous system and interferes with your body's ability to absorb vitamin B-12. So in a case such as this, daily supplementation of B-12 may make sense. In some cases of pernicious anemia, B-12 shots are indicated.

Most of the time a well-balanced diet satisfies most of your vitamin needs, unless your physician believes otherwise. Vitamin (and mineral) deficiencies often occur in elderly populations. Upon being admitted to the hospital for any number of reasons, large numbers of patients in their 80s and 90s are found to be undernourished, probably because of poor eating habits.

Vitamin D levels, in particular, are often low in the elderly, perhaps because of lifestyle patterns. Many folks in the over-60 crowd spend more time indoors than they did in earlier years, especially if they are infirm. Consequently, they don't get enough sunlight needed for the body to utilize vitamin D. (By no means am I recommending sunbathing.) In comparison to your diet of earlier decades, you and others in the Boomer generation may tend to eat decreased amounts of foods that are good sources of this vitamin, notably milk and milk products and fatty fish like salmon. Proper dietary regulation is vital at all stages of life, but adequate vitamin intake is especially important in older persons.

MINERALS

Minerals are nutrients also found in the food you eat. As with the case of vitamins, they contribute to healthful body function, and proper nutritional practice should guarantee an adequate supply of them. Some are required by your body in greater quantities than others and are known as *major minerals* (phosphorous, calcium, magnesium). Those that are needed in lesser amounts (less than 100 mg per day) are referred to as *trace minerals* or *micronutrients* (copper, zinc, selenium, and iron). Nutritionists continue to debate the relative importance of some of the so-called trace minerals.

Your body depends on minerals to satisfy two important purposes: to build skeletal and soft tissue, and to regulate vital processes such as heartbeat, blood clotting, oxygen transport, and nerve function. As you age your need for calories decreases, but your mineral needs are pretty much the same as they were when you were in your 20s and 30s, with vitamins D and B-12 being exceptions. In fact, you may even require more.

Whereas a certain amount of minerals is needed for proper physiological function, as is the case with vitamins, more than this minimum amount is not only wasteful, but also potentially harmful to your health. Some prescribed medications commonly used by persons over 60 may modify the way in which certain minerals are absorbed or used by your body.

For example, long-term use of antacids may result in copper deficiency, and other drugs used commonly by elderly persons to lower blood cholesterol may reduce the absorption of the mineral iron (exercise on the other hand, has the potential to reduce cholesterol without this negative trade-off). In such cases dietary supplementation of these minerals makes sense. But large and unnecessary doses of minerals can also prevent your prescription medications from making the contribution they should. That's why I strongly recommend seeking advice from your physician prior to embarking upon a program of mineral supplementation on your own.

You would be wise to consider dietary supplementation of minerals very cautiously. Don't fall prey to the television and magazine ads that promise miraculous benefits from dietary supplements without first seeking medical consultation to determine if you have mineral deficiencies. All too many claims about the benefits of minerals supplementation are lacking in scientific support. Don't throw money down the drain—be careful. In a nutshell, consider using dietary supplementation only when necessary. An appropriate question to raise at this point is, "Who actually benefits more from nutritional aids— the consumer or their manufacturers?"

Check out the website *mypyramid.gov*, an online interactive diet planning tool based on the dietary guidelines for Americans. All you have to do is enter your gender, age, height, weight, and activity level and you'll receive a suggested meal plan.

☞ WHAT YOU'VE LEARNED IN THIS CHAPTER

Very real and important connections exist among body image, exercise, and nutrition. Exercise can play a substantial role in body weight management and enable you to more closely approximate the physical appearance you desire, despite the influence of your inherited genes. Exercise can help you control your appearance. One of the outcomes of participation in a sensible exercise regimen is the elevation of your body's metabolic rate—the rate at which cells function—and therefore the amount of fuel they require. If you burn calories through exercise in excess of your metabolic needs, and keep your caloric intake steady, you'll likely lose stored body fat. This chapter explained how this happens and also discussed related concepts, such as hunger and appetite.

Foodstuffs, or the basic ingredients of what you eat, were also addressed in the chapter, in particular, water, carbohydrates, fat, protein, vitamins, and minerals. The relationship of these food elements to exercise, health, and well being were elaborated upon as well.

FOOD FOR THOUGHT	
1	Describe your appearance, as you believe others see you. Are you tall, heavy, thin, too thin, long of limb, broad-shouldered? What in particular do you like about the way in which you look? What would you like to see altered?
2	What can you do to change your appearance or any of its aspects that you don't like?
3	To what extent can exercise influence the way you look? Is an exercise program a realistic way for you to change your appearance?
4	In view of what you've read in the chapter, do you feel that your daily diet is proper? What kinds of adjustments might be in order?

Endnotes

1. 2010.
2. 2001.
3. 2001.
4. You, Murphy, Lyles, et al., 2010.
5. Romero-Corral A., Sommers, V.K., et al., 2008; Mahbubur, R. Berenson, A., et al., 2010.

Chapter 4

PSYCHOLOGICAL BENEFITS OF EXERCISE

What do scientists tell us about exercise and the mind? What exactly is *mind*? Is mind different than brain? Does the term *psychology* include both mind and brain? What's the connection between exercise and psychology? What are moods and emotions? Can exercise help us control them?

A Brief Comment upon the Discipline of Psychology

Psychology is the science of mind and behavior. It deals with such fascinating issues as learning, memory, emotions, and personality, as well as a host of other intriguing topics. In this chapter I propose to establish a connection between some of these topics and physical activity. I want you to appreciate the available opportunities for enhancing these dimensions of your psychology through exercise.

For about 50 years now, the discipline of psychology has been applied to the sport and exercise experience. This adaptation has emerged as a legitimate and valuable psychological specialty area. So much so that the venerable American Psychological Association now includes a division (Division 47) specifically devoted to sport and exercise. Many professional journals and organizations are dedicated exclusively to the interaction between psychology and physical activity. I and two

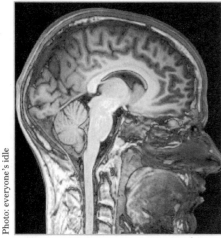

Photo: everyone's idle

Psychology is helpful in explaining what motivates exercisers, when exercisers stick with a program without quitting, and how rehabilitation from exercise injury can be facilitated.

of my colleagues, Drs. Bonnie Berger of Bowling Green University and Robert Weinberg of Miami University of Ohio, have written a book about this connection titled *Foundations of Exercise Psychology*, and I have produced four others of my own in this and closely related areas.[1]

Psychology is extremely helpful in explaining, among other things, what motivates exercisers, when exercisers stick with a program without quitting (see Chapters 7 and 8), and how rehabilitation from exercise injury can be facilitated (see Chapter 5). With the conclusion of these introductory comments, let's now turn to this chapter's intended target: physical activity's psychological pay-off.

As we age, some of our intellectual capacities lose vitality and sharpness. However, participation in regular, appropriately prescribed physical activity may slow these changes. An abundance of solid evidence exists in support of mental activities being improved through exercise.[2] As John Ratey, a Harvard University professor, puts it: "If you get your body in shape, your mind will follow."[3] It is this very link between exercise and psychological well-being that is of concern in this chapter.

The Psychology of Aging

ATTITUDE

Dr. Waneen Spirduso of the University of Texas, Austin, her colleagues, and graduate students have been systematically studying various aspects of physical activity in older persons for decades. One of her reported observations is that fit people tend to perform better on many mental tasks, especially tasks that involve speed and attention.[4] At the moment, we cannot conclude that fit Boomers necessarily have stronger overall mental capabilities than unfit counterparts. I wish I were able to assert that, but the available scientific research does not support the assertion. I can't promise you that the more exercise you do, the more pronounced will be your mental acuity.

What I can tell you is that a high level of fitness is associated with a slowing in the deterioration of certain kinds of mental abilities. And your attitude about aging can also have a vital impact on your psychological as well as your physical well being. Don't overlook this connection; it's important and real. But my telling you about this linkage is not enough. You have to buy into it. *You have to believe it.*

The more positive your attitude about getting older, the better will be your performance on memory tests. Older persons who hold positive attitudes about aging also tend to retain more of their hearing (a hallmark of old age) than those with more negative views. The will to live, being hopeful that your life is worthy and full, also correlate with length of lifespan. Aging itself is something that elderly persons dwell upon and worry about. Your attitude about getting older is a contributing factor in how well you actually age. Getting your mind off this process and maintaining a healthy perspective on chronological advancement is beneficial. Attempt to do so and bear in mind that exercise can help.

So what's the bottom line? Keep your chin up and your outlook positive and you may live longer. But be realistic. Be able to acknowledge that as a Boomer life is different than before, and there are undoubtedly some limitations to your achievements. You are entitled to feel a little anxious about some aspects of getting older. But strive to be as positive and optimistic as possible about passing birthdays. After all, what's the alternative to not getting a year older? Aging is an inevitable process, but it provides for some very savory benefits. And exercise is capable of optimizing these benefits.

Drs. Marco Pahor and Jeff Williamson comment upon physical inactivity in the January 25, 2010, issue of the *Archives of Internal Medicine*. Consider their bold and clear statement: "Physical inactivity is one of the strongest predictors of unsuccessful aging for older adults and is perhaps the root cause of many unnecessary and premature admissions to long-term care." Believe it!

You don't have to run marathons or bench-press 300 pounds. Just find a physical activity that's within your capability range, something reasonable and yet effective. Something that's in keeping with our aforementioned definition of exercise. I'm not pushing exercise craziness. I'm arguing in favor of something rational and safe. Take a look at the following newspaper excerpt that talks about what I consider to be excessive exercise, certainly *not* something that I'm recommending. The source is a Canadian newspaper called the *National Post*.[5]

George Herbert Mallory never made it to the top of Mount Everest. In fact, he died trying in 1924. But the ill-fated mountaineer did accomplish something by uttering three immortal words to a New York Times reporter that have been echoing down the valleys of human adventure-seeking ever since. Asked why he wanted to climb the Himalayan monster, the bright-eyed-soon-to-be-expired-young Brit replied: "Because it's there."

Contemporary adventurers seem to be testing more extreme limits than ever before: ultra marathon running across heat-blasted African deserts, cycling through war-torn nations, unicycling in the high Andes, solo sailing across frothy seas, tandem rowing across untamed oceans and running, always running—like never before. Take Stefaan Engels as Exhibit A. Mr. Engels ran a marathon in Montreal on Tuesday. It was not his first. He also ran a marathon on

Saturday. And Sunday. And Monday. He has completed a marathon a day, every day for 207 straight days. The plan is to keep on running until he hits 365.

Brain Change

Not only does your brain change during aging (it becomes smaller), but also the nerves that transmit messages to and from this vital organ operate somewhat slower and less efficiently than when you were younger. Parts of your nerve cells, called *axons*, are coated with an insulating material (*myelin*) that prevents the escape or diffusion of the electrical messages being transmitted. During aging this protective covering loses integrity, the same way that the rubber or plastic insulation on the wire that connects your table lamp to the wall socket deteriorates over time.

Brain wave patterns reflect this gradual deterioration, and those of older persons are different than those of younger people. Exercise seems to delay such age-related changes in the nervous system and thus the thinking and problem-solving capability of its command center—the brain. Older exercisers do better on many problem-solving tasks than those who are sedentary and therefore not as fit. So here you have yet another reason for engaging in regular physical activity; avoidance of slowdown in nervous system and brain function.

Exercise and Cognition

According to an interview with Dr. John Ratey of Harvard University,[6] in addition to maintenance of a healthy brain and nervous system, other mental health benefits come with regular exercise. This is not surprising because mental activities are reflections of your brain's health. The brain is an anatomical structure, and mental processes occur in this superb organ. Some brain functions are basically chemical and electrical, while others predominantly involve feelings or moods. Exercise naturally increases the concentration of important brain chemicals that stimulate the nervous system, namely *dopamine* and *norepinephrin*. These chemicals in synthetic form are of-

ten prescribed by physicians in cases where patients have difficulty in concentrating upon important environmental stimuli.
Exercise provides this outcome naturally.

Your brain is responsible for activities that involve thinking,
remembering, and solving problems. Scientists refer to these
functions with the term *cognition*. As I pointed out before, exercise seems to have a very positive influence on this process.
For instance, some recent research tells us that regular walking
is associated with a reduced risk of *dementia* (essentially a condition involving compromised cognition) in elderly men (see
Chapter 4). And tension, depression, feeling down, and fatigue
are reduced immediately after a bout of exercise. This has been
amply demonstrated in many studies.

In older persons who have been diagnosed with relatively serious (clinical) depression or anxiety issues, exercise reduces the
severity. Older exercise participants also report positive short-
term changes in self-concept, body image, and happiness after
a workout. I'm not perfectly sure why these effects occur, but
one way to explain them is that during exercise there is a tendency to be distracted from stress. Exercise enables you to disengage from troublesome stimuli and thoughts. Change in location may also be a contributing factor.

EXERCISE USUALLY REQUIRES VENUE CHANGE

More often than not, exercise necessitates a change in physical
environment. You can't swim, play golf, garden, or jog in your
kitchen or living room. If you have a very large living room,
folk or square dancing is a possibility, but usually exercise
means leaving the house. It may be that this change in venue
takes you away momentarily from factors that contribute to
your tension or anxiety.

A second possible explanation is that during robust physical
activity your body produces certain chemicals (in addition to
ones already mentioned), like beta-endorphins, which are
known to elevate moods.

A third explanation may relate to satisfaction with having
executed certain exercise or sport movements skillfully. If you
really played well, upon leaving the tennis court you feel ful-

filled and uplifted even if you lost the match. If you've walked your two-mile neighborhood course in a minute less than you usually do, the satisfaction puts a smile on your face. You feel uplifted. You feel better about yourself.

Satisfaction and positive mood change can also result from mere participation in vigorous physical activity simply because you know you've done the right thing: You've done something that's good for you. Even if the exercise made you tired, even though you pushed through it with a measure of discomfort, you've done it and you are pleased with yourself. Remember that feeling derived from finally finishing a difficult homework assignment in high school? You did it. You finished it. You completed something you were supposed to do. And you feel pleasure by virtue of having put it behind you.

Don't misinterpret what I'm saying. Exercise doesn't have to be unpleasant. What I'm suggesting is that a substantial dose of pleasure can be derived from nothing more than completing your bout of physical activity. And this satisfaction can transcend, or at least be an additional element to, all the other beneficial outcomes so far delineated (and more benefits to come).

One more point along these lines: When you enter an exercise environment—a gym, a pool, a jogging trail, a squash court—you put yourself in a place inhabited by others who value the same kind of physical activity as you do. In other words, you are in "good" company, company that sees things the way you do. In and of itself, this factor contributes to your satisfaction.

BODY IMAGE

Body image, or the view you have of your physical appearance, is a very influential aspect of your psychology. Exercising regularly over an extended period of time, typically, or at least very often, results in a change in body weight, especially if the exercise has been of the aerobic kind. If you've been swimming, walking, or jogging for a few months, you most likely have reduced the amount of stored fat in your body. This weight loss will be obvious when you examine yourself in the mirror, and as a result, the image that you've held previously about your body may undergo positive change. You like your body more. Because body image is an integral part of your entire psychology, when it shifts in a positive direction it has the potential to influence your overall psychology, your behavior, and the way in which you interact with others. The ways in which you evaluate your body very significantly influences the manner in which you think about your entire self (*self-image*).

COGNITION

Activities such as thinking, remembering, learning and utilizing language, making judgments and decisions, and solving problems are all part of the mental experience known as *cognition*. We humans do these things remarkably well in comparison to other species. Your brain, an absolutely incredible organ located within a protective rock-solid skull, is in charge of all your thoughts and emotions. But the brain also manufactures an assortment of very important chemical messengers that are distributed to various body tissues and organs so that they may carry out their important cognitive responsibilities. Exercise increases the volume, as well as the specific ingredients, of these chemicals.

Cognitive activities occur in your brain at highly specialized locations, each with a well-defined responsibility. Certain brain areas mapped by scientists, and actually seen with magnetic imaging, X-ray, or CT scans, are involved in short- or long-term memory. Others handle visual and sound discriminations. Mathematical manipulations and various kinds of puzzle solving tasks are dealt with in still other brain locales. All of these functions fall within the domain of *mind*.

Think of *brain* as an anatomical entity, a mainstay and executive command center of your nervous system. It's an organ—something that can be touched by neurosurgeons, examined visually and, when necessary, altered. Understand *mind* to be the working or thinking part of your central nervous system, the part that actually reasons, the part that develops your thoughts and ideas and executes your cognitive operations. Your mind is invisible. Unlike your brain, it cannot be photographed or seen, but the manner in which it functions can be trained and changed. This is exactly what teachers, parents, psychologists, and psychiatrists try to do.

The science of psychology is generally devoted to the study of mind and to understanding, predicting, and changing the visible behaviors that it orchestrates. Neuroscientists study brain anatomy and chemistry, and psychologists are concerned with our thoughts and physical actions.

Your brain's functional efficiency tends to decrease somewhat as you age. But fairly recent research published in the *Journal Trends in Cognitive Science*, a publication obviously dedicated to cognitive processes, offers the following welcome conclusion: Physical activity enhances cognitive and brain function and protects against the development of neurogenerative disease.[7] In a more recent publication (2009) the same authors, Kramer and Erikson along with others, report a significant association between fitness and performance on certain memory tests—those having to do with special challenges.[8] They discovered that among their elderly subjects (ages 59–81), those with higher fitness levels had a larger *hippocampus*, a brain part known to be vital in forming memories. So, if you can maintain a high level of fitness as you age you can retain valuable learning and memory functions—two important indicators of your quality of life.

These kinds of exciting findings beg the question: Why would you not at least attempt to find some form of exercise that you could call your own? Brain health benefits are yours for the taking. Exercise can be a cheap way to maintain or improve your cognitive functions. Don't discount such a valuable opportunity. Grab it! And if I'm wrong, the worst case outcome would be an improvement in your strength, endurance, flexibility, agility, and respiratory efficiency. You have nothing to lose.

COULD OLDER MEAN BETTER?

Gene Cohen, a scholar and scientist devoted to the topic of the elderly mind, in his groundbreaking book, *The Mature Mind: The Positive Power of The Aging Brain*, argues provocatively that our brains may get better as we age.[9] But even if Dr. Cohen's controversial thesis is not entirely accurate and some deterioration indeed occurs with aging, in healthy persons such change occurs very gradually. As you get older you tend to become a little more forgetful and probably a bit slower in your reactions to the constant barrage of environmental signals that demand your attention.

Fortunately, other factors that accompany aging may counteract these deficits. One such compensating factor is the vast number of experiences you've collected in so many different contexts during your lifespan. The game of tennis can provide an example. At age 65 you may not move as well as a teenage opponent who is just beginning to play. But over the years you have acquired court know-how and an acute understanding of the game's nuances. Years of playing and resulting court sense enable you to quickly assess your opponent's vulnerabilities and recognize the style of play and strategies she employs. In a nutshell, you've seen it all, or at least you've seen much more than the teenager facing you. What's more, you are tuned-in to your own physical capabilities. You know how to pace yourself on the court. You know when and how much energy and effort to expend, and you have a pretty good idea of what your youthful competitor is up to. The teenager may cover the court better, but nevertheless, not be a match for the savvy, psychological ploys, and self-confidence that derive from your years of tennis.

You know who you are and what you can do, and you simply go about doing it. The inference in this tennis example is also transferable to many other settings. Your vast store of past experiences can enable multitudes of advantages and successes in so many exercise as well as non-exercise areas. It's one of the wonderful benefits of transitioning into Boomerhood and beyond.

Hanging on the wall of my flute teacher's music studio is an adage that both informs and amuses me. It tersely summarizes my point: "Old age and treachery will overcome youth and skill."

OLD AGE AND THE PROCESS OF AGING

Psychologists use traditional milestones when referring to different age groupings. In so doing, they suggest that if and when you are able, or in later years, perhaps unable to accomplish certain physical and mental tasks, you thus graduate from one developmental stage to another. However, sometimes nothing more than age is used as a criterion or turnstile.

For instance, when a man is 45 he is labeled middle-aged; when he hits 70 he's old; when a boy is 16 he's still a kid, despite the fact that in almost every state he can be licensed to drive an automobile. These conventional designations are nothing more than matters of convenience, and terms such as *infant*, *youth*, *adult* and *elderly* are often applied loosely and inconsistently. They may be entirely incompatible with the view you have of yourself. Although you may have actually lived for 70 years, you may not consider yourself to be old at all. If you are satisfied with life, happy most of the time, and enjoy a high degree of wellness (see Chapter 2), irrespective of your chronological age, you are not old.

If you remain in control of your life and are pleased by the direction it has taken, this contentment entitles you to disregard the label *old*, regardless of the number of years you have lived. Being 12, 22, 32, or 42 years of age, in and of itself, does not guarantee happiness. It is your readiness to meet the physical challenges before you (your physical fitness status) that will dissuade you from feeling old. And frankly, if you are concerned about getting older, then by all means lead a physically inactive lifestyle which will certainly encourage more rapid aging. Of course you are older than last year, but not necessarily old. For sure, older individuals may have goals that are different from young people, but when personal goals are attained at any age, the result is fulfillment and great satisfaction.

At what age is one permitted to drive in your state? Is it the same age required for purchasing alcohol or enrolling in military service? The criteria for these adolescent milestones are different even in the very same state. So what does it mean to be a child or a middle-aged person? And what exactly is adulthood?

AGING

Consider aging as a process described by a horizontal line or continuum. At one end (the far left) we'll locate the newborn and call this point #1. At the other end (far right) we'll place people who are approximately 100 years of age and call this location point #3. If you are located at either of these extreme ends of the continuum, namely points #1 or #3, you are definitely not middle-aged. You are either very young or very old. However, if your location on the continuum is close to point #1, you are young. If you're located all the way to the right, or near point #3, then you are elderly. Point #2 represents middle age. Chances are that if you are reading this book, your location on the horizontal line is somewhere between points #2 and #3. But do you really care? Are these designations important or are they trivial?

Developmental psychologists are scientists who study characteristics in people who differ according to their location on our continuum. They are interested in differences in the way people think, what they think about, how they learn, and how they experience emotions. *Emotions* are feeling tones such as anger, fear, or anxiety. They are of brief duration, whereas *moods* are feelings that linger. For instance, you can be sad or extremely happy for an entire morning before you undergo a mood change.

For scientists who investigate these things, it is convenient and helpful to attach names to the various stages of development. They therefore use terms such as *infancy* (birth to one year), *early childhood* (1–5 years), *youth* (approximately 5–11 years), *adolescence* (not necessarily defined by age, but by ideas and issues that persons in this category must address and resolve), *adulthood* (the period between adolescence and older adulthood), and *older adulthood*.

The term older adulthood presents definitional problems that may be more troublesome than other stages of development. Experts disagree. Some consider this period of development to begin at age 55, while others believe that it begins at age 60, 62, or 65). A New York City bus driver will permit you entrance to the bus at half fare (senior citizen fare) if you show your Medicare card, which you acquire at age 62. And speaking of such discounts, perhaps you've noticed billboard signs that encourage you to stop for dinner or a night's rest at a particular restaurant or motel. Upon stopping at these places you discover that eligibility for the senior discount varies from one place to another. At one facility 55 years of age qualifies you for the special treatment; at another, 65 gets you the discount. You soon realize how capricious and arbitrary these designations are.

EUPHEMISMS AND LIMITATIONS

Writers and speakers who are fearful of alienating or offending their audiences often refer to persons of advanced years with substitute phrases. They use euphemisms, terms considered to be relatively less disagreeable, and avoid words such as *old* or *elderly*. Among these substitutes are: *senior citizens*, *seniors*, *old timers*, and *golden agers*. But many of us find such references to be offensive. I, personally, have an aversion to *senior citizen*. It leaves me with the distinct impression that I'm being patronized, and I don't like it. I would just as soon be called elderly, or better yet, an older person.

BE IN TOUCH WITH YOUR PHYSICAL CAPABILITIES

Compiling a list of what you can no longer do well or easily should not be too difficult. Your current capabilities are certainly known to you and you can readily identify activities that are simply not good for you or are too challenging. Without doubt you are in touch with your limitations and carefully and responsibly pursue daily activities with these in mind. Good activity choices are based upon an understanding of exactly where you are in your physical development as a person.

As I've already suggested, the process of development also entails a change in functional capacities. But remember, *you* choose the manner in which to be active. You may receive advice from others, but the final decisions are yours alone. Truth be told, we are not able to run as fast or as far as we could some 45 years ago. Some of us may not be able to remember things as efficiently as we did when we were young adults, and we certainly can't cover the tennis court as we did some 20 or 30 years ago (forget about basketball or baseball). But as long as you know who you are and what you can and what you cannot or should not do, you'll be fine. No one cares that you can't run as far as you used to. What is important is that you commit to a regular, sensible, made-to-order program of exercise of some sort. That's what's critical .

Although it is not especially difficult to list things you can no longer do easily, things that are now difficult for you to do, it is much more of a challenge to identify activities that you can indeed accomplish. What are your authentic capabilities? Now that you're older, what is it that you can safely do? What kinds of physical activities are surely in your repertoire at this time? The fact that all of us has a different status makes these questions difficult to answer. Nor is there general agreement as to what constitutes an *elderly* person. The term *elderly* covers a lot of territory. As already noted, different criteria are used in different contexts to define the term. A few years ago my uncle Charlie passed away at age 102 when I was almost 70. So he and I were both *elderly* men at the same time, despite a difference of more than 30 years; both elderly, but in reality not in the same developmental stage.

The changes that accompany all points on the aging continuum eventually occur to every one of us. But they happen at different rates, degrees, and times. This is precisely why it's not easy to generalize answers to the questions I've just raised to all so-called elderly men and women. The answers are person specific. Your authentic physical capabilities and your declared doable or not doable activities and movements are not the same as those of other readers of this book. However, almost all of the Boomer and beyond generation members can anticipate certain changes. But these unavoidable transitions and alterations bear upon your physical rather than psychological abilities.

AGE-RELATED PSYCHOLOGICAL CHANGES

As you age, you change, and when establishing a program of regular beneficial exercise it is important to understand your limitations, that is, the limitations imposed by aging. Only with such insight will you be able to construct and maintain a safe and effective routine. Let's now take a look at some of the changes normally ongoing in your bodily systems, those that particularly relate to your psychological function. And let's put them in the context of exercise. Some of these changes you might have already experienced, and others you may be undergoing now as you move forward age-wise and developmentally.

CHANGES TO THE NERVOUS SYSTEM

Your brain and nervous system contain basic units or cells known as *neurons*, which communicate with one another by chemical/electrical messages. The three basic parts of each and every neuron are the *cell body*, *axon*, and *dendrites*. The nerve impulse or message travels from the cell body along the neuron's axon en route to the hair-like terminal projections of the dendrites. From these small, thin projections at the end of each neuron the chemical/electrical message is transmitted to the dendrites of another neuron. The actual transmission occurs at a location known as the *synapse*. Strings of neurons, never actually touching one another, but nevertheless, in touch with one another, form *nerves*, which carry instructions throughout the body and tell your organs to execute their particular missions.

However, as you age the structure of the axon tends to change. Some of its fibers become tangled and withered, which results in the weakening or blockage of nerve impulses. Sometimes *plaques* (fatty blobs) clog the axon's fibers and inhibit the movement of the chemical part of the message (known as *neurotransmitters*). With less powerful communications occurring among brain cells, functions such as thinking and remembering are compromised. This also means that your muscles, for example, are receiving relatively weaker signals than they did when you were an adolescent or young adult.

As you continue to age, some, but not all of the dendrites shrivel and die. Some continue to grow during aging, but the entire communication mechanism is simply not what it was during your earlier years. Weakened messages to muscles results in slower contractions and reduced expression of power.

Your muscle tissues themselves also undergo changes over the years and therefore their capacities for contracting against loads is reduced. All of this is a consequence of aging.

But not to worry. You've still got plenty of capacity. You can still think, remember things, lift things, move well, and participate in sensible physical activities. However, it is essential that you thoughtfully and responsibly select activities that are appropriate for your less efficient but certainly still quite capable and proficient nervous system. You can certainly "move it, move it" but not with reckless abandon. You'll be pleased to know that exercise has been shown to increase the number of dendrites in rats, mice, and dogs, and researchers are presently working toward similar findings in humans.

CHANGES IN REACTION TIME
(HOW QUICKLY YOU RESPOND)

When it comes to finding complex targets on a computer screen, those over 60 don't do as well as adults under the age of 25. Performing more than one task at a time is also more difficult for those over 60 than for much younger persons, especially if the tasks are new. If you are scrambling eggs you are still able to pay attention to the music playing on the radio without difficulty because both activities are relatively simple. They require only minimal nervous system involvement.

You are slower than when you were a young adult when it comes to locating targets (attending). No surprise, and really no problem if you play tennis or bowl with people of similar ability. When you think about it, you may realize that many forms of physical activity do not make exceptionally strong demands on your ability to focus only on relevant or important cues. Walking or swimming, for example, do not require doing more than one thing at a time. After deciding upon exercise activities that are appropriate for you, try and locate partners or competitors against whom or with whom you can participate and who are of comparable skill, motivation, and enthusiasm. In doing this, you level the playing field, maximize your enjoyment and satisfaction, and reduce the probability of injury.

Older people take longer than younger ones to respond to stimuli. That is, you probably don't get off the mark as quickly, which may create the impression that some of your movements are impaired. This is not the case. You are not impaired in the strict sense of the word, but because you respond a little more slowly, it may appear that way.

But here's gratifying news: When you do respond your reactions may be more accurate than those of younger persons. In other words, you may very well be a better decision-maker if for no other reason than you have been making decisions for many more years than 20-year-olds. You are simply better at it because you have more experience. Furthermore, when given the chance to practice, you usually close the reaction time gap between yourself and younger persons. Bear in mind that wrinkles have nothing to do with reaction time or cognition.

CHANGES IN WORKING MEMORY

Holding onto information that derives from some prior experience (something you've seen, done, or read about before) in order to solve an immediate problem, answer a question, or decide between two things relies upon your working memory. Unfortunately, this kind of memory declines as you proceed into advanced adulthood.

This explains why you walk down the hall to the bedroom and then can't quite recall why you set out to do this in the first place. Your compromised working memory (also known as *short-term memory*) is the culprit. You were unable to hold onto thoughts that deal with your motivation for going to the bedroom. Somehow whatever prompted you to target the bedroom as your goal has slipped out of your awareness.

Three different kinds of memory exist. The first two are familiar: *simple recall* as when you remember a detail, name, or fact; and *recognition*, when you choose a correct answer from an array of choices. Everyone is prone to a memory glitch from time to time, but older persons tend to exaggerate such errors and worry about them. If you believe that your memory is strong you'll work harder in memory tasks. To the contrary, if you believe that age is depriving you of mental acuity you'll more readily fall prey to the notion that age is taking its inevitable toll.

The third kind of memory is *long-term memory*, or the ability to store facts, thoughts, names, etc., from yesterday or yesteryear. It stays intact much longer and does not weaken as a consequence of aging. You are thus able to pull up memories from your youth with little difficulty. You can regale neighbors and grandchildren with stories of your long distant past, although you can't quite remember why you are walking down the hall en route to the bedroom. Try not to worry about this. Laugh it off unless a thorough examination by your physician indicates that your ability to process information (putting information into the brain and then retrieving it for practical use) is abnormally compromised. If your memory is problematic, there are techniques you can acquire that will assist you in processing information. A book that can be helpful in this regard is by Spirduso and Poon. It requires somewhat heavy reading, but give it a try. Particular sections deal expressly with what we're talking about here.

By all means, realize that even though your memory might not be as strong as it once was, you still retain the capacity to remember, to process information effectively, choose wisely, and reason clearly. So what if much younger acquaintances can accomplish some of these mental operations a little better? Why not enter partnerships with them and harness their acumen when faced with recall or recognition challenges? They'll be delighted to collaborate because your greater experience in problem solving and patient reasoning will benefit them as well.

EXERCISE AND MEMORY

Results from an impressive array of research indicate that among elderly subjects, those who exercise regularly do better on tests of short-term memory and general information processing than those who are sedentary.[10] Once, scientists believed that such findings were due to training that resulted in increased blood flow to the brain. Although this explanation has been revealed to be untrue, the real causes of this phenomenon remain elusive.

Truth be told, I remain unsure why elderly exercisers fare better on memory tests, but they do.[11] So besides smiling at occasional memory lapses and acquiring techniques that assist in avoiding them, why not permit exercise to help? Decent evidence exists that cognitive impairment and dementia among elderly men and women may be prevented or its severity reduced with exercise.[12]

In addition to all of its other very legitimate benefits, exercise may very well be the memory strengthener you've been looking for. I believe that in this respect it's at least as good as any pill or elixir you can find on your pharmacist's shelf. Exercise is able to strengthen important brain circuitry and this potentiality may account for its positive influence upon cognitive function.[13]

Along these lines is an additional and fascinating connection involving regular exercise and the fearful, devastating medical bully, Alzheimer's disease. An article in *The Archives of Neurology*[14] presents data that suggest a link among muscle strength, Alzheimer's disease, and cognitive decline in older people (average age 80.3 years). Interesting. The more muscular strength you have, the lower the likelihood of cognitive decline as well as a lower probability of developing Alzheimer disease. One objective and potential outcome of exercise that I've elaborated upon in Chapter 1 is muscular strength. Here we are able to see yet another implication for its cultivation, especially in older persons.

Social Psychological Benefits of Exercise

Much more is involved in human psychology than cognition and personality. One other compelling specialty area is *social psychology*. I would be seriously remiss if I failed to relate exercise to this psychological subdiscipline.

Social psychological issues revolve around interactions with others—that is, from psychological perspectives. Social inter-

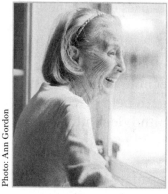

Are you intro-
verted, or do you
participate in
group exercise?
Social psychology,
or interacting with
others, can greatly
impact the mind
and body.

course is the balm, nourishment, spark, and fire that enables our lives to be both satisfactory and even more importantly, satisfying. Accounts of reclusive individuals who avoid or even shun the presence of others are widespread, and all of us have either heard of or know such persons.

Some people tend toward inwardly directed behavior, or as psychologists who study personality would say, toward *introversion*, but most of us thrive or at least are comfortable with our daily intermingling with others. Of course, there are occasions when all of us prefer to be alone. Well adjusted Boomers with high degrees of wellness are comfortable with most of their interpersonal relationships, although all of us can undoubtedly identify some folks whose company we can do without.

Participation in a program of regular exercise can foster opportunities for new acquaintances and sustain and strengthen those already formed. If your preferred form of exercise is participation in a team or individual sport, others are needed as teammates or opponents. If your preference is for swimming or jogging, walking, golf, bocce, or bowling you can't help but come face to face with others of comparable skill or enthusiasm for the activity. Swimmers share space in the pool and locker room; walkers and joggers greet and are greeted by like-minded exercisers. A smile or a "Good morning, nice weather" suffices as a primary contact on the track or road.

The next time the jogger, walker, or swimmer is encountered, the smile and greeting is warmer and less hesitant. A week or two later, upon seeing the fellow exerciser, you observe that she was absent from the scene the previous week and then learn she was out of town visiting a son and daughter-in-law. "Oh, how nice. Where do they live? Really, I'm familiar with the area. I've been there many times." And so on and so on. The same scene can be witnessed at the gym, YMCA locker room, or golf course clubhouse. If you are a tennis or badminton player you require at least one person on the other side of the net. If doubles is your game you need a partner and two opponents. Arrangements are necessary. Telephone calls must be made. You have to deal with people.

In other activity domains, opportunities to socialize are available but not necessarily mandated. Garden clubs exist for avid horticulturalists whose members spend hours planting, feeding, and caring for their plants and vegetables. Toward this end their physical engagement can be formidable and undeniably qualifies as exercise. They work hard. But they gather to chat about their pursuits and achievements. They trade techniques, successful methods, and secrets. They interact.

Leagues, in which bowlers and shuffle boarders congregate and compete, exist and attract fellow enthusiasts. Square dancers, ballroom dancers, cloggers, and tap dancers can't possibly pursue their passion without interacting socially as well as physically with partners or fellow participants. Sailors are often attracted to regattas where they meet others with identical or overlapping interests. Weekend t-shirt walks or jogs are on the recreational calendar of most communities and are advertised in local newspapers. Tournaments for tennis players and golfers and serious competitions for all sorts attract participants over 60. In Chapter 10 I'll enumerate national and international competitions in almost every conceivable sport.

So you go, you join, you do, you talk with other men and women. You establish contact. You get to know, like or dislike people. You interact socially and the contact is precipitated by your involvement in physical activity. True, acquaintances may be fostered through recreational activities that are devoid of the rigor and gross physicality that I'm recommending—of course. Bridge, bingo, and chess offer similar chances for social interaction. But others have probably written books about the virtues of such activities. I leave it to them. My business is exercise.

More often than not, exercise gets you out of the house,

which increases the likelihood of meeting and mixing with others, some of whom you may really take a shine to. It's even fairly probable that your social skills may be burnished as you acknowledge a need to cultivate friendships with people with whom you've had little prior experience. You acquire the sport- or exercise-specific jargon necessary to enter dialogue with other aficionados. You learn to talk about "sets" and "reps" in the gym, "pace" and "mileage" on the road or track, "flip turns," "stroke recovery," and "pushing off" in the pool. *Exercise offers exceptional opportunities for interacting with other people.*

☞ WHAT YOU'VE LEARNED IN THIS CHAPTER

In this chapter we've talked about the various age categories that cover life from birth to old age. I've attempted to explain what it means to be elderly and repeatedly made the point that age categories, although often convenient, are somewhat arbitrary in their designations. I for one am not enamored of certain euphemisms commonly used to refer to people who are advanced in years. I prefer to be thought of as an older man or an elderly man rather than a senior citizen or golden ager. I'm okay with being old as long as I understand the nature of the limitations that guide my behavior and as long as I feel comfortable accommodating them. Of course, you are free to ask persons in your immediate world to call you what you wish. Or you might determine that you really don't care one way or the other. What is important is that you come to terms with being older.

You've also been exposed to in this chapter to the ways in which your nervous system responds to aging and how inappropriate it would be to expect it to function as efficiently as it did when you were decades younger. Special emphasis was placed upon memory and the ability to pay attention as you continue to age. The nervous system, although somewhat compromised as you age, nevertheless is capable of very adequate activity. It will continue to serve you well if you understand that it is not what it used to be. And lastly, you learned that exercise could meaningfully contribute to the maintenance of the nervous system and its various operations. No surprise.

Lastly, the subspecialty of social psychology was introduced. In addition to the enumerated psychological benefits that entail neurological strength and cognitive function provided by physical activity, profitability of a different kind was discussed. The social opportunities offered through exercise were emphasized.

FOOD FOR THOUGHT	
1	Look in the mirror and ask yourself whether or not you have attained old age. Are you young elderly, elderly, or old elderly? Are you comfortable with what you've designated?
2	Identify changes that you've observed during the past few years in intellectual performance. Is your memory as strong as it used to be? Are there recognizable deficits in the ways you perform mentally? Describe the ways in which you try to compensate for these identifiable changes. Are you troubled by the changes you've identified?
3	Do you see a connection between exercise and maintenance of nervous system function? Describe this relationship to the best of your ability. Speak with your physician about this connection and seek further clarification.
4	Are you able to relate to the notion that exercise provides wonderful opportunities for developing new relationships? Can you envision such opportunities that may enhance your quality of life?

Endnotes

1. Foundations of Exercise Psychology, Berger, Pargman, &Weinberg, 2002; Physical Fitness: A Wellness Approach (2nd edition), Greenberg & Pargman, 1989; Stress and Motor Performance: Understanding and Coping, Pargman, 1986; Understanding Sport Behavior, Pargman, 1998; Psychological Bases of Sport Injuries (3rd edition), Pargman, 2007.
2. Paterson & Warburton, 2000.
3. 2009.
4. Spirduso, Francis, & MacRae, 2005.
5. http://news.nationalpost.com/2010/09/01/stefaan-engels-runs-a-marathon-a-day-every-day-207-and-counting/
6. Medscape Psychiatry and Mental Health (October 8, 2009).
7. 2007, p. 348.
8. Kramer & Erikson, 2009.

9. Cohen, 2006.
10. Report of the Surgeon General, 2010.
11. Gerda, Roberts, et al., 2010.
12. Lauern, Verrault, et al., 2001; Larson, Wang, et al., 2006; Ravaglia, Fortaluci-cesare, et al. [n.d.]
13. Kramer, Kirk, & Erikson, 2007.
14. 2009.

Chapter 5

AVOIDING EXERCISE INJURY

Peggy's grandson has been injured often while playing high school football. She had been fearful this would happen and had advised her son and daughter-in-law not to permit the boy to participate in what she considers a brutal physical activity. Her attitude may be summarized by her all-too-frequent comment: "What does he need it for? There are so many after-school clubs and organizations to keep him busy. Why does he have to take such risks and perhaps ruin his body forever?" Peggy's entire perspective on sport and exercise had been tainted by the spate of injuries experienced by her beloved grandson. When her physical therapist recommended she undertake daily walking as therapy for her advancing osteoporosis and arthritis, her response was adamant: "Exercise is not for me. See what happened to my grandson?

Peggy's naysayer attitude is ill conceived. True, some form of injury is not unheard of in physically active persons, but it is absolutely not an inevitable outcome. It doesn't have to happen. Injury is not a good thing no matter how you slice it.

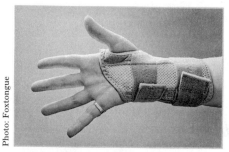

Photo: Foxtongue

Have no fear: if you design an exercise regimen that is sensible and safe, you can avoid the dreaded injury.

Understandably, when undertaking exercise one of your most important objectives is to reduce its probability. But if injury does occur, its consequences can be minimized. By making sure that your physical activity regimen is sensible and compatible with your abilities and needs, and predicated upon realistic goals, you can proceed with an exercise schedule with an intensity that is suitable and safe. In many important ways you are different than others—even different from those in your own age group. You therefore require, no less deserve, custom-made exercise prescriptions. If you permit good judgment to prevail and if you are in touch with your capacities, you need not face injury.

A DEFINITION OF INJURY

What exactly is injury? Does the term mean the same thing to everyone—physicians, athletic trainers, laypersons, physical therapists, sport coaches, and athletes? Actually, agreement is lacking, which makes it tough to write about injury definitively. When I use this term in my professional lectures or writings I give it the following interpretation: "Injury means trauma to the body or its parts that results in at least temporary, but sometimes permanent, physical disability and inhibition of motor function." This suggests that when you sustain injury, you are debilitated to the extent that you are unable to function as competently as before. If you should be injured as a result of doing exercise, my hunch is that at least one of the following five factors is culpable.

1. Inappropriate exercise prescription

2. Faulty execution of movement

3. Psychological factors

4. Subconscious factors

5. Environmental factors

INAPPROPRIATE EXERCISE PRESCRIPTIONS

You should not be doing certain movements or activities in the first place. Combative sports are inappropriate for most men and women over 60 years of age and the same probably holds true for contact sports like soccer and basketball. I say this despite my previous comments about self-concept and body-image and despite the widespread and enormously popular aphorism, "You are only as old as you believe you are." If you are 70 years old but feel like 60—terrific. But your joints, bones, and connective tissues have, nonetheless, been doing their awesome jobs for seven decades. Be fair to them.

If pain or discomfort occurs while, or soon after exercising, ask yourself, "Why am I doing this particular movement or activity? Who told me to do it? Where did I get the idea that this exercise is good for me?" Don't stubbornly proceed in a way that doesn't feel right. No virtue is found in being a martinet. Don't force yourself to execute certain movements or actions because a friend is doing them. Don't arbitrarily copy from others.

FAULTY EXECUTION OF MOVEMENT

An activity itself may be appropriate, but if you are doing it, or some part of it, improperly or inaccurately you may be a candidate for injury. You may have too much weight on one leg; you may be moving too fast; you may be struggling against too much resistance; you may be doing too many repetitions or sustaining the movement too long. When your body or any of its parts moves improperly (faulty mechanics), the erroneous movement results in inappropriate forces upon your bones, muscles, and connective tissues and is a precursor to injury. My recommendation is this: If you are embarking upon a new set of physical challenges, seek instruction. Find an experienced, competent person who can show you how.

Psychological Factors

Sometimes something of a psychological nature is causing mechanical interference with your movement execution. Perhaps it's fear or anxiety about what you are doing or planning to do. Maybe your self-view is exaggerated and inaccurate, and because it's incompatible with at least one of the requirements of your chosen activity, it is difficult to concentrate on related demands and requirements. Somehow these necessary movements trigger unsettling memories. And so your focus is off. You are oblivious to important environmental cues, or you don't process them properly. You therefore execute incorrectly and—bingo—you hurt yourself. Although you are not psychologically prepared to proceed with the activity, you engage in it anyway. What would be helpful in such circumstances is for you to pinpoint these thoughts, identify the psychic troublemakers, confront and deal with them—or withdraw from the activity all together.

Some of us are high risk-takers and enjoy a challenge with a modicum of physical danger. Others are at the very opposite end of the *risk-taking* continuum; that is, we have an aversion to behaviors that are even moderately dangerous. So if there is a mismatch between what a particular activity demands in terms of risk and your natural psychological tendencies, you'll be uncomfortable and turned off. Fertile grounds for injury. Be careful to consider what past experiences indicate about your risk-taking inclinations and project them to the activity's requirements. Be in touch with your risk-taking comfort zone.

A Word to the Wise

We all know someone of Boomer vintage who is still boxing, wrestling, playing flag football, hockey, or basketball. And some of these diehards participate quite credibly and, apparently, safely. But don't use these folks as models. These are people who have probably maintained high levels of fitness over the years or who are specially and generously physically endowed. They are exceptions. And most likely, if they had not been fitness devotees for long periods of time and not structurally and organically gifted, they would not be able to perform those types of activities. You may admire them and by all means wish them well, but don't emulate them.

An exception to my caveat would be participation in contact or combative sports that have been modified to accommodate your changed and changing physiological systems (see Chapters 2 and 4). Each year a handful of men and women well into their 80s compete in our nation's well known annual marathons: New York, Boston, Chicago, and others. These participants are not good prototypes for you to imitate. Be careful, prudent, and cautious. If your motivation to compete in combative or contact sports is irrepressible, then at least make sure the playing field is level. Compete according to age group.

If you are interested in a psychological perspective of sport injury you might have a look at a volume I edited titled *Psychological Bases of Sport Injuries* (3rd ed., 2007). For this project I invited 20 prominent researchers and scholars to each contribute a chapter. Although the book is not focused on elderly persons or those of the Boomer generation, I believe you'll find some interesting and helpful ideas and commentary.

Subconscious Factors

Things bubbling in your subconscious mind are causing trouble. They are inaccessible albatrosses around your neck that pick away at you. But you don't know or understand why. They are deeply buried, murky, and unavailable to deciphering without professional assistance. These memories and thoughts defy your interpretation, yet they somehow interfere with your ability to attend to important and helpful body signals. These cues serve as guides for safe and appropriate exercise behavior, but since they are now compromised, your muscle and limb actions are false or inaccurate. And so you incur injury. Sometimes these psychic irritants operate in ways that inhibit safe and accurate movements, thereby setting the stage for miscalculations, missteps, and injurious consequences. Trust your instincts. If you have a hunch that a certain activity is not right for you, even if you don't understand why, avoid it.

Dr. Burt Geiges, a friend, colleague, practicing psychiatrist, past President of the Association of Applied Sport Psychology, and an admirably smart guy to boot, has recently put forth a new professional website (http://www.nurtgiges.com). It's worth pulling up and reading. In presenting his "Philosophical Perspectives" he comments upon a point I'm addressing here. Admittedly, he's mostly referring to athletes who are, or were, his patients and not necessarily members of the Boomer generation. But what he says is applicable to all of us. Here's a bit taken from his website. Think about what he says in reference to injury prevention and exercise. Try to relate his message to my brief treatment of subconscious factors.

> The focus of my work with athletes and others is to help them change those patterns that contribute to distressed feelings or troublesome behavior, and to remove the barriers to their optimal functioning. This focus is primarily on present experience, based on the hypothesis that past negative experiences might recede into the background, were it not for the fact that present patterns of thinking and feeling keep them in the foreground. The language used by the person is followed very closely, because it not only expresses present thoughts and feelings, but also contributes to their development. I believe that what we learned in the past can be changed by what we learn in the present.

Environmental Factors

Injury can also result from improper decisions about when and where to exercise. When you put bravado before common sense and disregard nasty weather conditions in order to exercise out of doors, you increase the probability of injury. Icy or wet surfaces make for slippery footing. Postpone activities such as jogging, walking, and cycling under such conditions. If winter, outdoor activities are your cup of tea, dress wisely. Hands and feet should be protected with gloves, mittens, warm socks, and appropriate footwear. Because a very large portion of body heat is lost through the scalp, (heat escapes through the many tiny blood vessels in the scalp), make sure that your head is covered. Take care of those ears as well—you have but two. Their lobes can be frostbitten when unprotected. Skiers and ice skaters pay attention.

Rain-slickened outdoor surfaces are precursors to slipping and falling, and slipping and falling set the stage for injury. Failure to acknowledge important environmental considerations may lead to injury. Injuries are not always caused by accidental events. They are often the result of carelessness, failure to abide by common sense, or blatant irresponsibility.

SOME GENERAL PRINCIPLES AND GUIDELINES TO HELP STEER YOU CLEAR OF EXERCISE INJURY.

1. Don't overdo.

    Rest between exercise days, and rest immediately after exercise. This doesn't mean lying in bed or even being seated. If you are jogging or running, intersperse a little walking between laps or miles. It's okay. A change in physical activity is also a legitimate interpretation of rest. Ride your bicycle one day, walk the next. Work in the garden one day and swim the next. Take a day off now and then, just like big-time athletes do.

2. Despite my previously offered cautionary remarks, if you've hitched your wagon to someone you know and are using him or her as a model for exercise, be certain this person's needs, health status, lifestyle, and motivation for exercise parallels yours as closely as possible.

    What's good for the goose may not be good for the gander. Select exercise and physical activity models cautiously. Highly skilled and experienced exercisers make an activity or movement seem easy. Don't be misled by their grace and accuracy. You may not yet be ready to follow suit.

3. Acknowledge sensations of pain and discomfort.

    Don't be a hero at the risk of injury. If something hurts, stop. Mild discomfort may be acceptable, particularly in the early stages of your program. But don't fall into a vanity trap—it's perfectly all right to stop if you're in pain.

Pain is a warning that something is wrong. Nerves that carry pain messages are located all around your muscles. When muscle tissue is compromised—even slightly—your brain knows about it and tells you so. You feel it.

4. When exercising out of doors adjust to environmental conditions by acknowledging them and complying with what they require. Dress appropriately, drink plenty of water, etc.

Drink before and even during exercise. Most of your muscle tissue, as well as all other tissues, consists mostly of water. Most of blood is water. During heightened metabolism exercise-induced elevated body temperature, your supply of cellular water is decreased and should be replaced. Don't rely on the sensation of thirst. By the time you feel thirsty during rigorous physical activity, you may be seriously water deprived.

ANOTHER WORD OR TWO ABOUT OVERDOING

Too much of a good thing can create problems. In order for exercise to be effective and benefit your overall health and physical fitness, it must be done regularly at appropriate levels of challenge. I've said this on a few occasions. However, this mandate gives rise to the question, "How much is too much, and how much is too little?"

A schedule that is too ambitious will increase your vulnerability to injury. But a routine that falls short of challenging your body's various physiological systems will not enable you to accomplish your health and fitness goals. So shoot for three workouts a week. (My answer to the question, "How much?") A fourth may be in order after months of participation—when your muscular, skeletal, and cardiovascular systems have strengthened and made necessary adjustments.

Be sure to take into consideration social, family, and professional commitments. The inveterate golfer, jogger, cyclist, or gym habitué who places exercise above family, social, and even perhaps career commitments jeopardizes the smooth rolling of the wellness wheel we considered in Chapter 2. Your lifestyle should accommodate a variety of interests, each deserving recognition and attention. Exercise is but one aspect. The wellness and contentment I spoke about in Chapter 2 will not come easily if a single dimension of lifestyle is overpowering. The idea is to establish and secure balance and not become so dedicated to your exercise program that it overshadows other dimensions of life. Once again, a word to the wise should be sufficient.

One of the most common causes of exercise injury is overuse. It is important that you provide your muscles an opportunity to recover from their efforts. During vigorous exercise muscle fibers tear a bit. This is not a cause for concern because they are capable of self-repair after rest. In fact, when these microtears are repaired your muscle function is improved. The ability of your muscles to overcome resistance is thus enhanced. They become stronger. This is why it's important to provide rest between workouts and why I say that three or possibly four days a week is not only sufficient, but also preferred.

When overused, muscles may incur damage that goes beyond microtearing: Damage that will self-repair with a day or two rest or damage that could have been repaired with rest, but none was forthcoming.

When muscle tissue is subjected to repetitive stress without sufficient time for healing, the resulting injury is usually due to *overuse*. But this kind of vulnerability is not restricted to your muscles. Your bones and tendons are also susceptible. A very simple way to understand this term is to say that overuse involves *doing too much*, with the consequence being excessive tissue breakdown, which is problematic. When the demands of your physical activity exceed your physical abilities or your readiness for challenging effort, the result is overuse injury. *Be smart; be cautious; be realistic; be safe. DON'T OVERDO IT!*

SOME EXERCISE-RELATED INJURIES

At first I had trepidation about including the following section for I was concerned it might dampen your enthusiasm for what I'm so lavishly praising. If my descriptions are too lurid and vivid they may be disconcerting to the extent that they turn you off and divert you from exercise. But I eventually concluded that a very brief and light discussion of possible negative exercise consequences might serve two desirable purposes. First, it might ratchet up the degree of caution you would apply in building and implementing an exercise plan. And second, it might ease the psychological burden that accompanies exercise injury, in the event that it does occur.

If injury happens, you will at least understand what has transpired biologically and what may be in store. My wish is that by abiding by the cautions and advice offered in the paragraphs above, you will significantly reduce the likelihood of injury. Moreover, it's entirely possible that you may never be victimized by exercise injury (although it may indeed happen).

A little education about medical terms such as *muscle strain*, *muscle contusion*, and *stress fracture* (known as *traumatic injuries*), as ominous as they sound, should be helpful. If nothing else, an understanding of what's involved in each condition may provide a platform for comforting a friend who has suffered exercise injury and who would benefit from your knowledge as well as your compassion and sympathy. I'll emphasize *preventive measures* that you can take to avoid injury rather than discourse on what should be done remedially. I leave such discussion to physicians, physical therapists, and other medical personnel. One other point: Unless you plan to participate in combative sports such as rugby, soccer, or football (and you realize from my prior comments that I advise against it), broken bones are not strong probabilities.

My assumption is that most folks over 60 years of age are not likely to enter such forms of physical activity. Muscle damage of some sort is one thing. Bone trauma is something else entirely. By the time we reach 60, bone density has significantly decreased in comparison to what it was during our 20s, and females lose density sooner than males. Therefore, even without exercise or sport-related assault to your skeletal system, as you age, fractures remain a concern. As we get older, tissue in joints also tend to change, which may lead to arthritis or similar conditions. These changes create susceptibility to injury in joints, bones, and connective tissues.

Not everyone beyond 60 is afflicted with osteo or rheumatoid arthritis (which by the way are not the same in terms of their causes), but those who are should seek advice from physicians in order to be sure that the physical activities chosen for exercise are suitable. This is an additional example of what I mean when I say that the activities you choose for your program should be consistent with your personal needs, interests, and capabilities. I might add that it is certainly not unusual for a physician to prescribe some form of physical activity or exercise for an arthritic patient.

You have more than 300 muscles in your body—a good 50% of your total body weight—and they are used continually throughout the day. During exercise the resistances against which they must function are significantly increased, and they are often called upon to contract against loads that are well above their typical challenge. But you'll be gratified to know that your muscular system is capable of withstanding a considerable amount of stress before it succumbs.

Having made this point let me continue by saying that when a muscle is stretched excessively during physical activity *muscle strain* may occur. Muscle strain is a partial tear or damaging stretch in the muscle. The muscle becomes hard or knotted and very painful. Swelling and bruising may appear in the area over the few days following injury. You'll certainly know when and if a strain happens. If the muscle tears entirely the term *rupture* applies. Insufficient muscle strength and flexibility are contributing factors to strain and rupture.

STRETCHING

Muscle injuries are probably the most common of all exercise-affiliated traumas but by no means life threatening. One problem with addressing injured muscles is that it is often difficult during everyday living to provide the immobilization and rest that they require for healing. They'll usually heal by themselves if you can avoid re-injury. A good body of scientific evidence suggests that warming up and stretching the large skeletal muscles before exercise helps prevent injury, although some debate continues as to whether running speed is actually improved with pre-performance stretching. (But our issue here is injury prevention, not speed.)

A warmed muscle that has been stretched before the demands of exercise have been imposed is far less vulnerable to strain or rupture than an unprepared muscle. This benefit is probably due to one very important objective of the stretch, namely improving range of motion. Moreover, warming up and stretching increase your muscle's elasticity and blood flow.

Some experts suggest that *dynamic stretching* is best before aerobic exercise; and *static stretching* is best after exercise. Dynamic stretching represents an attempt to replicate the movements of a particular activity. For instance, if you are preparing to swim, you would move your arms in a manner that mimics the swimming motions. But after the swim workout, you would stretch the muscle group statically: You'd hold the stretch for about 20 seconds or until you no longer feel strong tension in the muscle or muscle group.

Pilates is an exercise format that involves very controlled movements and strengthening of the body's *core muscles* (abdomen, lower and upper back, hips, buttocks, and thighs). It also emphasizes *body awareness* or knowing where the body and its parts are located in space.

Yoga is a form of exercise essentially concerned with improving strength and flexibility. It utilizes poses or postures performed slowly and quickly. In my view both yoga and Pilates should be supplemented with some sort of aerobic exercise in order to ensure a comprehensive approach to fitness. Advocates and practitioners of yoga speak highly of its capacities to improve balance and reduce stress and anxiety.

A FEW THINGS TO REMEMBER WHEN STRETCHING:

1. Try to isolate the muscle or muscle group that you wish to address. Consult an anatomical chart that indicates which muscles are to be involved in your chosen physical activity and its major movements.

2. Stretch gently and slowly. *Do not bounce while stretching.* Hold the stretch for about 20–30 seconds and then gradually release it.

3. Stretch to the point of mild tension. *If you feel pain STOP!* Overstretching can cause damage to muscle tissue.

4. Don't hold your breath while stretching. Breathe naturally through mouth and nose.

5. Try to increase the stretch slightly each time you do it.

An excellent reference to consult if you wish to learn more details about stretching is *The Stark Reality of Stretching: An Informed Approach for All Activities and Every Sport*, by Steven D. Stark (4th ed., 1999).

Muscular contusions are bruises caused by severe blows or falls. Banging into another exerciser, falling on a hard surface, or being struck by an exercise or sport instrument such as a baseball or cricket bat, tennis racket, or snow shovel may result in muscle contusion. Blood vessels are ruptured, which causes discoloration of the skin atop the afflicted location. The area becomes black and blue, which, I suggest with tongue in cheek, can become some sort of a prideful indication of your being an avid sport or exercise participant. Prideful badge notwithstanding, contusions also bring tenderness and pain.

STRESS FRACTURE

Fracture refers to a break or crack, and although I suggested previously that unless you are engaged in heavy contact sports such as football or soccer, the probability of being afflicted by this condition is low. *Stress fracture* is another story altogether. Here a singular, significant trauma or blow to a bone is not the cause, but a cumulative or built-up overuse or stress on the affected part of the skeletal system.

Stress fractures develop over time, usually in the weight-bearing bones of the lower leg and foot. They show up as thin lines on X-rays. Walking or jogging for months on end with improper footwear or on surfaces that are inappropriate or abusive is often a contributing factor. Select footwear carefully in order to prevent this problem. Choose shoes that accommodate your particular foot characteristics. Don't try to save money by buying cheap exercise shoes. In the long run you'll pay a hefty price. Check the heels of your exercise shoes and look for signs of wear on either side. *Pronation* or rotating your foot inward and downward will tend to show wear on the inner margin of the shoe. If you are a *supinator* your shoe will show erosion on its outer margin because you tend to rotate your foot outward and upward when you move. Exercise shoes with wide (for pronators) or arched lasts (for those who supinate) can be helpful.

COMING BACK AFTER INJURY

Let's say you've hurt yourself during exercise. You were on your knees gardening and as you reached to pull a handful of weeds you pulled something in your back instead. Or your swing on the fifth tee caused something to go awry in your shoulder. Owwww! Consequently, you're out of commission for a week. Perhaps you struck a stone or tree root with your big toe while walking briskly on your favorite trail, and it's been killing you each time you take a step. So you put your walking program on hold for a while in order to heal.

Now the pain has subsided, your back or toe feels much better, but you wonder if it's OK to return to physical activity. Should you pick up where you left off? Should you cut back for the first two or three times you exercise? How much should you back off?

First, you are to be congratulated on contemplating a return to physical activity. This is good. The fact remains that if you are engaged in fairly rigorous and regular exercise, sooner or later some sort of physical glitch may happen. If you are cautious and sensible this need not occur often, or when it does, the discomfort and setback will be minor and short lived. A good program of physical activity that is custom-made to your needs and level of preparedness should instill within you a desire for continuation. The activity itself should be pleasurable and the awareness of progress toward a high or higher level of fitness should be rewarding. As I pointed out in Chapter 4, your self-concept and body image change in positive ways as you become more flexible, stronger, and generally more fit. It makes sense that you'd want to return as quickly as possible to activities and routines that have enabled this improvement.

ON A PERSONAL NOTE

I've had my share of exercise-induced injury. I've sustained fractures of various kinds on more than one occasion. With hindsight's benefit I realize that each and every injury—one or two of which were quite substantial—involved irresponsibility, poor judgment, or risky decision-making on my part. I knew better but made poor choices.

As I reflect upon what happened I'm certain that all of my mishaps could have been avoided. One discernable silver lining in my injuries is having learned that responsible, thoughtful decisions and good judgment are strong deterrents, and that competent medical advice will enable recovery. You can come back. You can return to your exercise routine after rehabilitation, healed and somewhat smarter and chastened.

Orthopedic medicine and its methods and technologies are nothing short of miraculous. Damaged or worn out hip, knee, and shoulder joints are routinely replaced today by the doctor-magicians. My best guess is that the development of many of the orthopedic surgical tools and procedures was prompted by the need to rehabilitate elite collegiate and professional athletes as well as wounded men and women in the armed services. We older persons are beneficiaries because these techniques are also applied to body parts not necessarily damaged by injury but compromised through decades of nothing more than wear and tear. I have quite a few friends and acquaintances who are once again jogging, playing tennis, and tripping the light fantastic on the dance floor after successful joint surgery. These reconstructive and rehabilitative opportunities are available for qualified patients. Let's hope you don't have to avail yourself of them. At least not for quite some time.

One more word about recuperating from injury: Do what your physician advises. Apply the very same level of commitment and seriousness of purpose to your rehab program as you did during your fitness-oriented exercise regimen. Regularity and rigor are foundational to both endeavors.

Again, if you apply good judgment, take what I'm saying to heart, and use the common sense and multitude of lessons you've been developing and experiencing through decades of living, you should be able to avoid exercise injury altogether. But if you do hurt yourself:

- Take your time returning. Even if you feel ready, delay the return for another day or two. If you've been exercising regularly for months, your fitness base is probably elevated and secure. Don't worry about loss of strength or aerobic fitness if you've been out of commission for a few days.

- Upon returning to your routine, test the vulnerable body part with very gentle movements. Make sure there is no pain or significant discomfort.

- Cut your normal routine (resistance, distance, or number of repetitions) in half the first day of your return and see how it feels.

- If you still have discomfort, don't hesitate to stop and desist from further exercise for another few days. *You want to prevent reinjury.*

Your main indicators of readiness to return are the absence of pain, swelling, and stiffness in the affected area or areas. Consultation with a physician is really your best bet in order to get details about your injury as well as information about the appropriate time for your return to exercise. However, the general comments and cautions that I'm providing here should also be helpful.

If you use your injury to rationalize a complete withdrawal from your exercise protocol and thus decide not to resume, search your soul in order to determine whether or not the activities you chose were right for you in the first place. Perhaps your selection was the type of copycat choice we've spoken of previously, predicated on inappropriate modeling. Perhaps you entered a particular form of physical activity that was unfortunately wrong for you. And now that you are in discomfort you've decided to withdraw entirely. Rather than quit altogether, identify another activity that really suits you. Choose more wisely this time. *Don't give up on exercise.*

EXERCISE AND SOCIAL BENEFITS REVISITED

In addition to a multitude of physical benefits already described, regular exercise offers a host of psychological and social payoffs. We've talked about some of the psychological advantages of physical activity and the very worthwhile social benefits it offers in Chapter 4. But there's an injury twist that's worth mentioning here.

Meeting people, the precursor to establishing friendships, is facilitated through participation in a structured program of physical activity. You dog owners know this to be true. How many new persons have entered your life, even casually or briefly, as a result of conversation taken up during dog walking or exercising? The golf course, tennis court, swimming pool, skating rink, the dance floor at the local senior center, the walking trail in the park—all are venues for person-to-person interaction. We've talked about these benefits in the previous chapter. These are places where social contact occurs, or can take place.

Many of these activities are also associated with clubs or organizations wherein members extend their interests in physical activity to the purely social domain. What I'm suggesting here is that these social opportunities may also play a prominent role in decisions to return to exercise after injury. You miss your jogging or walking buddies, your bowling acquaintances, your tennis doubles partners, and the Friday evening dance parties. Exercise friends and partners may try to sustain their relationships with injured exercisers and find ways of integrating them into activities despite their being temporarily off their activity program.

One of the things sport psychologists highly recommend to trainers and coaches of injured athletes is that attempts be made to keep them somehow involved in team efforts and activities despite their temporary disability. Creative coaches find ways to involve their injured athletes. And injured athletes can attend team meeting, keep score during games, and help newcomers in acquiring new skills.

The same strategy applies to your exercise world. If injured, try to somehow remain part of your exercise community. If another person in your exercise group is injured, find ways to extend some sort of social support in his or her direction. Perhaps you've been victimized by a similar kind of injury and could share your experience, particularly the pathway you took to recovery and return to physical activity.

☞ WHAT YOU'VE LEARNED IN THIS CHAPTER

Exercise injury was the focus of this chapter. With prudence, insight into your own abilities and level of preparedness for rigorous and regular physical activity, injury may be avoided or the probability of its occurrence reduced. Overuse, or doing too much physical activity, was discussed and you were cautioned about its potential role in injury.

The term *injury* itself was examined and an overview provided of its common causes. You were also introduced to other terms: *muscle strain, muscle tear, contusion*, and *stress fracture*. These were briefly discussed to provide familiarity with their symptoms should they occur to you or another exerciser known to you.

Guidelines for stretching movements designed to reduce the probability of exercise injury were provided in this chapter. The importance of warming up prior to exercising was also discussed.

Yet another chapter emphasis was upon the social dimensions of exercise. Not only can social support be motivational in that it may stimulate commitment and participation in exercise, but it can be very helpful in assisting someone victimized by injury. Expressions of sympathy and concern, and inquiries about rehabilitative progress, go a long way in sustaining the patience and motivation necessary for following the physician's or physical therapist's therapeutic prescriptions for recovery.

You were also reminded on more than one occasion in the chapter to be careful about adopting exercise intensities, frequencies, and type that you've observed to be working well in others. Your very own needs, readiness, and abilities are essential considerations and not those of others.

FOOD FOR THOUGHT

1	What is the most important or helpful piece of information provided in this chapter—one that you believe would offer a decent protection from exercise injury if acknowledged and integrated into your exercise behavior?
2	Imagine that an acquaintance of yours—someone with whom you had been exercising regularly for five months—has sustained an injury that requires withdrawal from physical activity for at least three weeks. Specifically, what would you say to this person? How would you try to be helpful?
3	What's the message conveyed in this chapter about modeling? Is it that modeling is entirely inappropriate in the exercise domain?
4	Consider your own location—where you live and exercise—and enumerate special considerations that apply in terms of engaging in robust physical activity.

Chapter 6

EXERCISE AND STRESS

Scenario #1

Even though I always play with people I know and like, an hour or so before I'm scheduled to step on the tennis court I start getting nervous. My stomach starts to churn, and I can feel my heart pounding in my chest. I don't understand it. Everyone talks about how relaxing the game is, but for me it's stressful. The very idea of having to compete upsets me. When I play poorly I become angry and frustrated. Maybe I should give up tennis.

Scenario #2

Every morning I eagerly look forward to my walk. I can't wait to begin. My daily cruise in the neighborhood is the most invigorating and pleasurable part of the day and when the weather is inclement and I can't do it, I'm tremendously disappointed. The walk relaxes me and induces a calmness that I don't get in any other of my daily activities. During the three miles that I cover, I think more creatively than at any other time. Interesting ideas and solutions to problems come to me, and I thoroughly enjoy the feeling that I'm using my body in a way that it was intended to be used; that I'm doing something positive and healthful. I start feeling the uplift as soon as I begin lacing my sneakers.

So, which is it? Does exercise *induce* or *reduce* stress? The chapter opens with a discussion of stress, its causes and consequences. I introduce the provocative notion that stress may be positive as well as negative and that stress associated with exercise can be a good thing. I explain how this works; how physical activity may relieve stress symptoms but other types may actually induce it. I introduce the term *physiological arousal* and link it to exercise. I put you in touch with a term re-

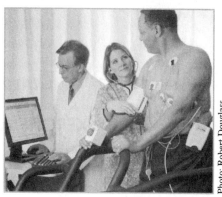

Exercise, when executed properly and consistently, can play a very large role in reducing bad stress, while promoting *good* stress.

lated to stress (but not the same), namely *anxiety*, and explain the important differences between the two. And finally, I recommend ways in which stress and anxiety may be managed or controlled.

What Is Stress?

Let me first suggest that a universally acceptable definition of this term is simply not available. As was the case with the word *injury* discussed in Chapter 5, scientists, writers, exercise experts, and psychologists differ in their interpretations of this complex concept. Let me introduce the term by presenting some background material that will ultimately be very useful in understanding the stress-exercise connection.

The term itself probably harkens back to the 17th century usage, which at that time referred to man-made structures such as bridges and edifices, and the loads they were expected to endure. Today, the term has important psychological implications, although it is still very much part of the civil engineer's vocabulary.

In my writing or speaking on the topic I refer to stress, very simply, as an unsettling reaction to events or factors occurring or having occurred in the environment. These factors, known as *stimuli*, represent changes in your internal or external environment (outside or inside your body). Loud noises that disrupt tranquility, for instance, or pain caused by inadvertent contact with a hot stove are examples of stimuli that you perceive as *stressors*. They are bothersome or disturbing, and you therefore respond negatively to the changes they cause.

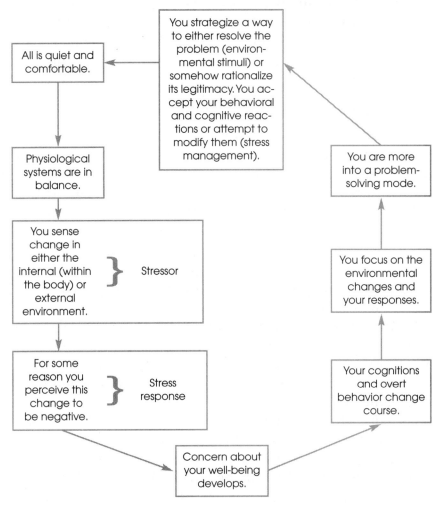

Figure 6.1. Stress response.

Stressors activate and alter your biochemistry, and depending upon their strength, can roil and rile your body's prior zone of comfort. The desirable physiological balances among your body's organs and systems, as well as their explicit functions, are knocked out of kilter. In sequence, your awareness of the biochemical/physiological disturbances initiates thoughts, feelings, and emotions. These, in turn, become additional stressors that charge and stoke your overall reactions. The words *perceptions*, *feelings*, and *emotions* are psychological and demonstrate the connection between mind and body. You burn your hand—it hurts—you emit a curse word or two, and your attention is directed toward doing something about the pain. You are distracted from your prior focus. Figure 6.1 represents this chain of events.

EUSTRESS VERSUS DISTRESS

But not all initial reactions to environmental stimuli are necessarily interpreted as negative or unsettling. Sometimes a change in body chemistry may have a positive overlay and desirable consequences. For instance, someone may say something that irritates you and so you retaliate with anger. Then you take action or behave in a way that has favorable results: You resolve a critical problem or you locate personal resources of which you were previously unaware. Your initial anger is the stimulus (stressor) that unsettled you, but the bottom line is positive.

Another example of how a stressor may eventually produce a positive outcome involves sexual arousal. During sexual stimulation your vital signs are in a dramatic state of psychological and physical upheaval. Your internal biological systems are completely out of whack. Your heart rate and blood pressure have gone haywire. But you are in seventh heaven. You are thoroughly enjoying your involvement. Some authorities use the term *eustress* as a way of expressing good stress, and *distress* as a reference to responses that are undesirable.

Stress, therefore, according to my clarification, is not necessarily a bad thing. And this is precisely what I meant when I remarked earlier that not all authorities agree on the best way to explain its causes or consequences. Many believe that whenever the word stress is used, there's invariably an implication of negativity or undesirability. I see things differently and later in this chapter when we broach the topic of exercise in relation to stress, I'll return to this point. I'll argue that although technically stressful because it initiates physiological commotion, exercise is good—very good.

One more relevant observation: Irrespective of the situation being eustresful or distressful, your internal and external physical responses are practically the same. Among the reactions to stress that you are capable of sensing are (not a definitive listing, but merely examples) a change in facial skin color, increased perspiration, increased muscular tension, increased respiratory rate, and increased heart rate. These responses are observable without medical training. You become aware of them. They occur in almost identical fashion whether your stress is due to pre-exercise fear and insecurity or to the exhilaration accompanying exercise. They are the same whether you are reacting to touching the hot stove or are in the throes of sexual excitement. However, the intensity of your reactions is likely to vary.

Alternate Ways of Understanding and Defining Stress: Some Brief Explanations

THE PSYCHODYNAMIC APPROACH TO UNDERSTANDING STRESS

Some authorities argue that the underlying causes of stress operate subconsciously, that memories buried deep in low levels of awareness become accessible when some contemporary trigger sets them off. These memories surface and stimulate psychological discomfort that is manifest physically. If these responses are negative or frightening, they cause physiological turmoil.

This understanding of stress is referred to as *psychoanalytic* or *psychodynamic* approach and was popularized by the renowned Sigmund Freud and his disciples. Psychiatrists and psychotherapists who undertake treatment of clients with stress disorders probe their subconscious thoughts, memories, and fears. The older you are, the more memories you've stored. And it follows that a full, varied, and rich collection of memories probably includes some that you interpret as unpleasant or negative. As a Boomer you've undoubtedly collected an impressive array of memories that lie under covers of dust, residing somewhere in one or another layer of consciousness. When that dormant experience is sparked into breaking the surface of the sea like a submarine, it carries the potential for psychic agitation. Why? Because it must be dealt with in the moment. It thus becomes a stressor.

THE LEARNING-ORIENTATION APPROACH TO UNDERSTANDING STRESS

Among alternative ways to understand stress is what I call the *learning orientation*. This approach suggests that the ways in which we react to stressors are acquired or learned. During childhood, parents, siblings, and perhaps movie and sport heroes demonstrate stress response behaviors that we inadvertently or intentionally integrate into our own way of doing things. As we age and move forward developmentally and chronologically, still other models continue to appear. And we emulate them.

We copy behaviors of friends, teachers, colleagues, and a host of others with whom we interact frequently. Acquaintances may tell us that we tend to fly off the handle easily, we are not patient, or we are admirably and enviably calm, cool, and collected. Hence we try to either change the ways in which we react to stress or comfortably and happily stay with a response mode that seems to work well for us and for which we are reinforced. But it is other persons in our environment who teach us how to cope with stressors. Figure 6.2 represents this way of conceptualizing stress.

THE PERSONALITY APPROACH TO UNDERSTANDING STRESS

According to some authorities, among them Dr. Charles Spielberger, emeritus professor of psychology at Florida Atlantic

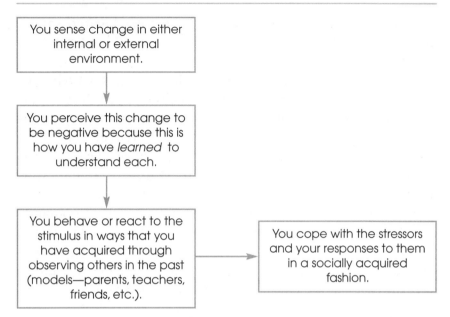

Figure 6.2. Understanding stress through the learning oriented model.

University, there resides within our very own collection of personality traits a predisposition to respond to environmental stress stimuli in a particular way. That is, we each have a certain behavioral style that defines us as individuals, and part of this personal behavioral style is the tendency to react to stressors in a prescribed manner. Spielberger prefers the term *anxiety* rather than *stress* and doesn't distinguish between the two. He maintains that we all differ in this trait and his paper and pencil *Trait Anxiety Scale* (1972) is used to determine its degree of strength.

Some individuals demonstrate substantial affinity for anxiety and are said to be highly anxious persons. They seem to be perpetually under the dark cloud used by cartoonists to suggest that one of their characters is in a funk. They are Gloomy Gusses because of their tendency to interpret surrounding events as problematic despite evidence to the contrary. Conversely, some of us test-out to be low in trait anxiety—the

"What, me worry?" type. And still others are located smack dab in the middle of the continuum and respond moderately to stressful stimuli.

Just as some of us are "naturally" shy, caring, nurturing, or introverted or extraverted, so are we inclined to confront stressors in a patterned fashion. We are not all provoked by environmental stress stimuli in like manner. Moreover, some psychologists believe that these variations may have a genetic basis or are at least partially influenced by genes. It appears that more and more of what we do or do not do as humans is currently being attributed to our genetic inheritance. Proponents of this controversial approach, known as *behavioral genetics*, suggest that our way of accommodating stressors is also genetically influenced. Behavioral geneticists are even now arguing in favor of a genetic basis for motivation to exercise.

SOCIAL/ENVIRONMENTAL APPROACH

Still one other way to clarify stress reactions is not through understanding necessarily what models you imitated but appreciating what is happening in your social environment at a given moment. Instead, what's going on your interactions with other people and what's happening moment to moment determines how you respond to stress stimuli. The emphasis here is upon the surrounding social framework. With whom are you speaking? Are you late for an appointment?

According to this way of understanding stress and stress response, social interactive stimuli are the only authentic triggers for stress reactions. The emphasis is upon the milieu in which you are functioning. What's important here is what others in your immediate social surroundings are doing to you or with you. Your interpretation of their current or potential influence upon your welfare determines whether you respond stressfully or not.

This brings us once again to the term *perception*. Perceptions are interpretations of events (stimuli) that are ongoing around us. And in this model the events are of a social (with others) nature. If you decipher current social events as potentially harmful or threatening then you are likely to respond stressfully. Particular factors, of course, may mitigate the intensity of your response, namely prior similar experiences and special characteristics of the environment. For instance, church, football stadium, physician's office, courtroom environments, etc., dictate whether or not sound stimuli (words, crowd responses) are acceptable, annoying, or stressful.

The point is that when you suspect that what someone is saying or doing is not in your best interest, then you react stressfully. This emphasis may be stretched a bit to include not only what other persons are doing but also things or props in the social environment that suggest or represent what others might possibly do. That's why the clock is a common stressor. It projects implications and assumptions about what other persons are doing or expecting. The clock tells us that we are late for an appointment. The clock tells us that we are spending too much time in the dentist's waiting room or that we are too early for dinner despite tummy grumblings. Think of Louis Carroll's rabbit in his *Alice in Wonderland*. He meanders through his scenes with watch in hand, constantly bemoaning his tardiness. He's stressed.

ANXIETY—NOT THE SAME AS STRESS

Although often used interchangeably with the word stress, anxiety and stress, in my view, are different. It's true that both often produce similar effects, but the processes that cause these responses have different dynamics. Anxiety is a form of fear, but not exactly the same as fear. When we use the term *fear* we recognize a concrete and identifiable element in the environment that undeniably threatens our safety. A weapon pointed at us is a fear stimulus. A grandchild rushed to the hospital in an emergency produces fear. The problem/stimulus is palpable; it's real, it's rational.

Anxiety is different in that an aura of uncertainty attaches to the event. You are not sure why you are upset. Something about this person or event fills you with doubt. You can't quite put your finger on what's bothering you, but you are troubled, worried, and apprehensive. You are anxious.

Anxiety is what you feel when you step onto the tennis court against a player whom you have beaten handily many times. Rationally, there's no reason for you to be on edge; ample evidence testifies that he or she is no match for you. But you are nervous about something and you are aware of your unease. You can't pinpoint exactly what it is, but you are jittery. Doubt gnaws at your innards. You pose an appropriate question but have difficulty answering it. You ask, "What am I worried about?" But you can't produce a legitimate answer. You are in the throes of an anxiety reaction.

Anxiety is a product of uncertainty about what's bothering you. The underlying causality is unclear, vague, or misunderstood. The hypothetical tennis player presented in Scenario One of this chapter's italicized introduction is under the influence of anxiety rather than responding stressfully. One of the nice things about exercise is that it favorably modifies the anxiety response. I'll return to this shortly and explain how it works.

Stress is different. When you are responding to a situation stressfully, the nature of the problem is obvious. And it's often of a physical nature. You know exactly what's upsetting you. You cut yourself while peeling potatoes; you dropped a prized piece of china; you were bitten by a prowling yellow jacket. You react to pain or disappointment, but the critical thing to remember is that the element of uncertainty is not a part of the experience. Not so in the case of anxiety.

Athletes and exercisers experience both kinds of responses—anxiety as well as stress—and each is accompanied by physiological arousal. Your body chemistry cranks up during either of the two reactions. When engaged in skillful activities, the efficiency or accuracy with which you perform are affected. The impact of arousal is often very significant. It sometimes benefits physical activity because some performances are improved by physiological excitement. But sometimes physiological arousal is a loadstone that worsens physical performance. An invigorated and significantly activated physiology, such as may be expected as a consequence of exercise, may produce either effect. Let me further develop this notion of how arousal or excitement may be helpful or unhelpful.

The Arousal–Performance Connection

If a skill is well learned, arousal is likely to be beneficial up until a certain level of physiological excitement. By well learned I mean a movement or movements that have been practiced diligently over time and which your neuromuscular systems can reproduce at will with accuracy and efficiency. But not all kinds of practice will yield positive outcomes. Just by repeating a movement over and over again by no means guarantees successful skill acquisition.

The practice must be done with diligence and insight, as is the case with any form of learning. Repetition alone will not hack it. Doing something over and over again doesn't necessarily beget a well-honed movement. In fact, practicing something repetitively can generate behaviors that are absolutely incorrect if the practicing is wrongful. Bear this in mind if your exercise preference depends heavily upon skill such as with archery, golf, squash, and dance.

Now back to the matter of arousal. Imagine a horseshoe standing on its feet, with its rounded portion on top. This upside down U represents a picture or graph of the relationship between arousal and performance. The very top of the horseshoe, where it curves or bends, is the location of your best performance. Either end of the horseshoe, where the feet are located, is where the execution of the skill is weakest in terms of accuracy, efficiency, and potential for error.

At one end the arousal is too weak; at the other, it's too strong. Skill execution or performance is lousy at both ends, where both feet of the horseshoe are. The idea is to determine the place on the upside down U where the amount of physiological stimulation is just right for you and for the type of exercise or skill you are attempting. Again, this best activation level is special to you and your particular activity. Your exercise companions may need more arousal than you for their best performances. And you in turn may require more than someone else you know.

The name of the game is to determine your very own optimal level of activation for a specific activity. Different activities and their associated skills require specific degrees of activation. And you get a handle on this by trial and error. Don't adopt another person's arousal level as your own. Remember, if you operate at an inappropriate arousal level you will probably sacrifice performance efficiency and accuracy. With decreased efficiency and accuracy you have to work harder to achieve desired results. This, in turn, opens the door to fatigue, disappointment, poor execution, or even all three. Thus, you operate at a deficit.

Your Optimal Level of Arousal

How can you determine your optimal level of arousal for a particular type of exercise? You do it on an intuitive basis. Bring to mind your best previous execution of a particular set of movements. Try to recall a time when your tennis serve was absolutely superb, when your putting was masterful. Try to remember how excited or aroused you were prior to, and if possible, during the activity.

- Were you especially calm before taking your putter out of the bag and lining up the shot?
- What do remember about your anxiety and arousal when stepping onto the court that day?
- Regarding your overall physiological stimulation—was your heart pounding and thumping rapidly?
- Were you perspiring heavily?
- Was there tremor in your hands?

These are signs of stress or anxiety reaction but may have nothing to do with temperature or humidity. Nor do they necessarily relate to your physical exertions and efforts. If you answer yes to all or some of these questions—it means that you were considerably cranked up or highly aroused due to psychological factors. And if your performance was really good . . .Bingo!

You should try to replicate or at least come as close as possible to the same degree of activation. Although psychological stimuli may be the underlying cause, you can manipulate your arousal level via physical means. This is one of the reasons that athletes warm-up before competition.

If you believe that you are underaroused (your arousal level is at the low end of the horseshoe) then do something about it. Either utilizes a psychological ploy such as bringing to mind an irritating thought or by briefly doing something physical that is activating (jumping in place). Athletes often jog a bit to increase arousal prior to competing.

Conversely, if you sense that your physiology is too highly charged, somehow reduce it. Fine tune it. Calm down. Take a few deep relaxing breaths or sit down. Some exercisers use headphones and recorded music to relax. Take and retake your pulse in order to ascertain that you've achieved a comparatively lower state of arousal. Although not always the case, usually low pulse equates with low arousal.

But bear in mind that the recommendations I've made in the past few paragraphs relate to skilled movements that are typically inherent in sport. If you are about to garden, walk, or swim with an emphasis upon recreation rather than competition, then arousal is likely to take care of itself. And therefore seeking the optimal level that we've been discussing is not of essence.

MANAGING STRESS AND ANXIETY
RESPONSES THROUGH EXERCISE

Recall that arousal means revved up physiology. The little cells in your body are like tiny factories. Each organ (heart, lungs, liver, and so on) chugs away at its own pace, fulfilling its destiny—doing what it's supposed to do. During stress or anxiety the pace is accelerated. The rate at which all of your cells operate in unison is referred to by the term *metabolism*, and your metabolic rate is higher when you are physiologically activated.

In and of itself, exercise is physiologically stimulating and can result in heightened metabolic activity to the extent that it is counterproductive. In other words, there's too much going on, physiologically speaking. When this is the case and your cells are generating a surfeit of hormones, chemicals, and waste products, the delicate biochemical balance that provides for emotional comfort is displaced. Thus, you feel agitated and disquieted.

But exercise can alleviate this irritability and discomfort (distress). Rigorous physical activity requires energy, and so metaphorically speaking, the body scans its available supply of chemical stuff, finds what it requires in various storage depots—the so-called surfeit mentioned above—and uses it. In this way the overabundance of body chemistry caused by stress is tapped and reduced. In this manner exercise burns off the extra chemistry accumulated as a consequence of the stress or anxiety.

Not surprisingly, exercisers frequently report feeling relieved of stress symptoms after a workout. They learn that exercise can be a way of managing stress. It is not uncommon for a person who acknowledges the presence of stress to announce that she is "going out for a jog"—a therapeutic jog, that is. Upon returning she reports a much improved frame of mind and attributes the change to her run. Punching the punching bag or chopping wood are clichéd remedies for managing stress and anxiety.

THE BRAIN DISENGAGES FROM WORRY DURING EXERCISE

One other very interesting hypothesis proposed by Dr. Arne Dietrich of the American University in Beruit attempts to explain how exercise is helpful in stress management.[1] Dietrich suggests that exercise may take the sharp edges off higher brain centers that are involved in anxiety-producing thinking (namely the prefrontal cortex of the brain).

In order to be responsive to the demands of exercise, the brain disengages from its worry mode and focuses on the requirements of the exercise. But it is now also obliged to deal with thoughts about fatigue and potential harm to the body, as well as any cues and alarms generated by the body in response to exercise. One caveat about this hypothesis: The exercise must be demanding and fatiguing if this redirected focus of attention is to actually occur. In keeping with this explanation, be mindful that a heavy bout of physical activity might reduce your anxiety and stress, but it can also be exhausting.

One more thing: Long-term exercisers tend to score lower on paper-and-pencil tests that measure trait anxiety than nonexercisers (we've already talked about Professor Spielberger's ideas). But—and this is a big BUT—when considering really strenuous bouts of exercise (think running or swimming hard), anxiety levels tend to rise and stay elevated for about five minutes post exercise. What this suggests is that your biochemistry needs time to settle down before anxiety finally decreases.

WHEN YOU EXERCISE, YOU TYPICALLY CHANGE VENUE

In addition to the explanations offered above (burning off excess physiology associated with stress and redirection of cognition or focus during exercise), another possible clarification comes to mind; a very simple one at that. If you are intent on addressing your stress through exercise, are you not obliged to change venue? You cannot jog or chop wood in your office, kitchen, or location wherein the stress reaction is occurring. The very act of relocating or removing yourself from the stressful environment may significantly contribute to the management process. Leaving the kitchen where a spousal altercation is ongoing may not be the best solution to resolving the dispute's core issues, but it may very well enable stress reduction. Leaving your desk loaded with bills, putting on comfortable shoes, and hitting the road for a brisk walk will not get the bills paid, but it may be an antidote for the distress associated with the mound of invoices and bills. Try it!

BEING OUT OF DOORS—IN NATURE— HELPS RELIEVE STRESS

Some decent evidence supports a case that being out of doors has an uplifting effect. According to Professor Richard Ryan of the University of Rochester's department of psychology, and colleagues, "Nature is fuel for the soul."[2] Exposure to nature correlates positively with an elevated sense of well-being and somehow repels or reduces feelings of fatigue. People tend to claim heightened energy when they exercise out of doors. Their moods seem to change in a positive direction.

Lastly, let me briefly mention a point I make at greater length in another book I've written. The book is titled *Managing Performance Stress: Models and Methods.* In it I write about another dimension of exercise that may contribute to the frequently reported beneficial mood changes associated with a regimen of physical activity that some years ago John Raglin and William P. Morgan at the University of Wisconsin labeled *the shower effect.* One of my graduate students, Jennie McGinnis, and I also observed this phenomenon in a piece of research conducted at Florida State University, where I taught before retiring. We realized that after exercising, most participants showered and changed clothes before being queried as to their mood. We concluded that this refreshing denouement of the exercise might be a contributing factor to the stress and anxiety reportedly decreased after the physical activity.

Having said all of the above about the potential of exercise in stress management, in order to be fair, it's necessary to flip the coin over and admit that exercise, when done with reckless abandon, when carried to excess or done improperly, may actually induce stress. Throughout this book I've hammered away at the need to exercise sensibly. Not surprisingly, overindulgence in a good thing can produce negative consequences and the same holds true for exercise.

The idea is to harness the power of stress and all the physiological activity it generates. Exercise can be helpful in this regard, but if you commit to an unrealistic program of exercise—meaning that the prescriptions you undertake are beyond your physical capacities—you'll compromise the entire strategy.

To be worthwhile, exercise should challenge you in many ways, but if the demands are extreme and you are incapable of meeting them, you'll burden your various systems (respiratory, cardiovascular, musculoskeletal, and so on) to the extent that you will stifle the desire to continue or consider future workouts with dread and trepidation. You'll create a stressful situation, with physical activity per se being the culprit.

Exercise Addiction and Dependency

When you exercise, in fact even before you start and are in a preparation mode, your brain signals various glands and organs to get ready. As a result, certain feel-good biochemicals begin to surge. Some of these products, known as *neurotransmitters* and *hormones*, have the capacity to calm and soothe. When exercise terminates, the levels of these chemicals subside and return to their more typical degrees of concentration in the blood and other fluids.

This is why some hardcore runners with years of running experience describe a sort of *withdrawal syndrome* when dispossessed of their regular run. When deprived of their run they become aware that the desired chemical infusion has not occurred. They miss it and sense the privation. Terms like *dependent* or *addicted* surface when referring to such phenomena.

I distinguish between the two: I prefer to view the actual chemical deprivation as a form of addiction—just as is the case with the removal of a drug (narcotic) from someone's life to which he or she relies upon for physiological well-being. I prefer to think of dependency as more of a psychological requirement wherein habituation has occurred. The dependent individual has become so adjusted to the comfortable feelings associated with exercise—the improved self view, the awareness of enhanced fitness, and elevated wellness in general—that a sense of loss prevails when deprived of the opportunity to exercise. In both cases the consequence of this deprivation may be stress and/or anxiety reaction.

Sport as Exercise

If we substitute the word *competition* for *exercise*, the picture changes. First of all, activities such as golf, softball, volleyball, and tennis, which obviously involve playing against others, may actually be stress inducing. The notion of competition itself brings to the table a need to master an opponent. Sometimes this necessity is subtly implicit in the athletic activity and sometimes it is blatantly expressed.

The word *competition* itself can't possibly be defined without somehow acknowledging the idea that an opponent exists. Competition is a social process and the word *social* connotes interaction with another or with others. Yet, the opponent of record need not be another human and may be inanimate, such as a mountain ski trail, a distance to be swum, or a number of yards, laps, or miles to accomplish on the jogging track. Something or someone must be vanquished if you are active within a sport context.

Sport exercisers understand that someone, some group of persons, or something must be beaten for the venture to be considered successful. Recognition of this requirement can be emotionally daunting or even frightening for some. Even elite athletes—those who are world class or recognized as national champions—report high levels of pre-, mid-, and post-performance anxiety and/or stress. To win is good; to lose is bad. Often these reactions are formidable and overwhelming. I've counseled such individuals and written about them in one of my other books, *Managing Performance Stress*.[3]

However, these aversive responses are not limited to sport participants. Among the men and women with whom I've worked are musicians (quite a few), public speakers, and other performers. These people frequently find themselves in authentic competitive circumstances. The demands of their performances involve confrontation with other persons or environments that must be bettered or conquered. But an effort that is perceived as valiant, effortful, sincere, and skillful might also be viewed as highly successful despite the scoreboard registering a technical loss. However, elite athletes are rarely appeased by the so-called moral victory. To qualify as a good boy or girl they must win, absolutely. Let me exemplify this alternate form of competitive success, the moral victory, by sharing a personal experience.

I WON

Some years ago I decided to run a marathon. I trained for months, abiding by all prescriptions of experts I knew. I did all the proper things. I established realistic and sensible training and performance goals (see Chapter 8). Goal number one was to run the entire 26 miles and 286 yards and not walk a single step. Goal number two was to complete the course in four hours or less. And goal number three was to awake the morning after the run uninjured and be able to walk the length of my driveway unaided. I reasoned that if I succeeded in satisfying these three goals I would declare myself a winner. I explained this to my three kids, and I lectured them about the essence of victory, its definition, and the various ways it could be interpreted. I was creative and utterly didactic. They heard me out with patience and doubt. I met all three goals. My devoted kids graciously awarded me a victory. I didn't come in first; scores of finishers beat me to the finish line. But I won.

DIFFERENT FOLKS,
DIFFERENT DEGREES OF COMPETITIVENESS

Trait psychologists tell us that personality profiles vary from one person to another. Some experts maintain that we all possess the same personality attributes but our individual endowments are highly variable with regard to their strength. Admittedly, some *personologists* deny the existence of traits altogether and attempt to clarify variations among our behavioral tendencies using alternative explanations. But those who are strictly invested in trait personality theory maintain that one of the attributes in our individual assemblages is *competitiveness*. Some of us are stronger than others and some of us are especially low in this trait.

Those at the low end are usually uncomfortable in situations that demand demonstrating excellence over another person or object. That is, they don't like to compete. When they are obliged to do so, they are likely to react anxiously and/or stressfully.

Conversely, those with particularly strong competitive tendencies seek competition, gravitate to it, and enjoy it. For such individuals the thought of competing is both energizing and inspirational. But the arousal is *eustress* in nature—the positive kind that we spoke of previously. They love to compete. They harness their loaded physiology advantageously and translate it into a more powerful golf swing, tennis groundstroke, or faster swimming pace. Their arousal is channeled into the performance itself.

It is common for exercisers who are involved in combative sports or events that emphasize explosive strength, such as football and weight lifting, to strive to elevate their physical arousal immediately prior to stepping onto the field of play. Such attempts are known as *psyching up*. They have learned that inflated degrees of physiological arousal will be beneficial.

This is in contrast to those whose sport requires relatively delicate movements such as pistol shooting, basketball free-throw shooting, or fly casting (fishing). Such activities demand a steady hand and relaxed muscles. Where are you situated in this scenario? Do you know persons who seem to be strong in trait competitiveness? Are you among them? Or do you prefer to avoid competition whenever possible?

The critical thing is to be in touch with your own propensity. You have been living with yourself for decades. Your self-knowledge is reliable and predicated upon hundreds of thousands of personal experiences. If the mere expectation of competition scrambles your insides, creates consternation, and is off-putting, it should not be pursued as a preferred form of exercise. If you err in this regard and choose to compete, the vital element of *exercise pleasure* will be diminished or entirely erased.

Instead, choose to rally with a tennis partner and don't keep score. Don't establish rigid or implacable weekly or monthly jogging or swimming goals because doing so places you in what is referred to as *indirect competition*—but competition none the less. In Chapter 8 we'll talk about realistic exercise goals, their importance, and how to go about setting them. I'll suggest that when establishing a personal exercise regimen it is critical to establish targets on a daily, weekly, monthly, and perhaps annual basis. However, if the goals are too challenging and unrealistic then the result is usually stress and anxiety. Be cautious.

In addition to differing in our need for or interest in competition, we also differ with regard to other personality characteristics. Some of us require more stimulation, more risk, more thrill in our lives than others. And so, at various levels of awareness we seek such experiences. You, for instance, may recognize a need for excitement and adventure that drives your decisions and behaviors .Others you know have learned over the years that their personal requirements for danger, risk, or stimulation are low. And so, in order to maintain a zone of emotional comfort they steadfastly avoid high levels of arousal. They routinely deflect adventurous and physically challenging situations. They are not likely to select rock climbing, scuba diving, parachuting, or paragliding as their exercise modus operandi. To each his own—the better you know yourself, the more wholesome, the more safe, the more appropriate will be your exercise decisions.

If you're the kind of guy or gal who finds competition exhilarating and highly motivational, if you thrive on the need to conquer a situation or someone else, be aware that sometimes the person against whom you compete may be none other than yourself. If this is who you are, then by all means consider sport as your primary form of exercise. But remember, a wide array of exercise choices is available to you. You don't have to compete in order to satisfy the need to be physically active. Any physical activity done improperly or excessively can induce anxiety.

So know who you are. Look to past experiences and your responses to them and choose activities wisely. Rigorous physical activity is typically and necessarily stressful to a certain extent because it places heightened demands upon your physiological systems. But it need not be accompanied by the harassment, worry, and overall dissatisfaction associated with anxiety or stress. Chapter 9 will help you make appropriate exercise choices.

OTHER WAYS OF HANDLING YOUR STRESS
AND ANXIETY REACTIONS

I've made a case for exercise being a good way to manage stress
and anxiety and attempted to qualify this recommendation. By
no means does exercise stand alone as an exclusive strategy, although as you can imagine, I endorse it as an efficient, readily
available, nonmedical way of managing stress. It's one of my
preferred approaches and I, of course, encourage you to consider it the same.

Here's a list of time-honored ways I'm unable to delve into
here, but about which you can read at your leisure in references that deal with stress in more general terms.

1. Behavior management techniques

2. Hypnotherapy

3. Massage therapy

4. Music therapy

5. Aroma therapy

6. Humor therapy

7. Muscle relaxation techniques

8. Biofeedback

9. T'ai chi

10. Mental imagery

☞ WHAT YOU'VE LEARNED IN THIS CHAPTER

The focus in this chapter was upon a phenomenon known as
stress. Implicit in all that was discussed was the notion that the
physical activity inherent in exercise may itself be stressful.
The term stress continues to elude definitive definition, and experts are not in agreement as to what it actually means. To different authorities stress conveys disparate understandings.
These differences were reviewed as were a number of essential
elements of the concept that experts seem to agree upon.

You were encouraged to consider stress a response to environmental stimuli that you interpret as being potentially threatening. The way(s) in which you react to these stimuli are the same, irrespective of the nature of the stimulus. Whether the threat has to do with imminent danger to your general health, the need to perform in a forthcoming competitive experience, meeting financial obligations, or an ear infection, the observable symptoms are essentially the same—increased breathing, heart rate, and perspiration, as well as many changes in body chemistry. Exercise may be a cause for a stress reaction, especially when performed incorrectly or in excess.

A distinction was made between stress and anxiety. The latter was described as having an element of worry, insecurity, and a vague understanding of how the environmental stimuli pose a threat to well-being. In the former case, stress, the source of discomfort is understood and might not be considered threatening at all. For example, you may be walking rapidly or jogging and thus respond to the demand stressfully. However, you interpret this reaction as being good. Observable stress and anxiety reactions are virtually the same; however, their causal underpinnings are different. If you are wired to devices that assess various aspects of your physiological arousal, the expert deciphering your data will not be able to pinpoint its nature or causes. The reviewer of your printout can only conclude you are experiencing stress or anxiety.

Competition, by definition an element of sport, may, in and of itself, be a source of stress or anxiety. The idea of confronting another person and attempting to defeat him or her, or demonstrating mastery over a physical obstacle (a mountain to climb, a descent on skis, or a prescribed distance to swim) may trigger stress responses. Therefore, choose your form of exercise carefully. Faulty decisions about how to exercise or how much to exercise may precipitate stress and anxiety.

Don't lose sight of the fact that exercise, in order to be helpful in the various ways discussed in Chapter 4, should be rigorous and physiologically activating. Be prepared to experience stress when you exercise, particularly when you partake of the aerobic kind.

	FOOD FOR THOUGHT
1	What temporary changes in your body are you able to recognize when you feel stressed? Do you respond stressfully in the ways enumerated in this chapter? Of the physical symptoms described, which seem to operate most dramatically in you?
2	Do you believe that you have strong competitive tendencies? Do you like to compete? Do you enjoy exercising in a group setting or are you more comfortable being alone during physical activity?
3	Have you ever experienced stress relief via exercise? When in the throes of stress have you ever resorted to an exercise solution? What was the result?
4	Do you agree with the premise that physiological arousal due to stress may be used to improve exercise performance? Can you provide testimony in support of this contention?

Endnotes

1. 2004.
2. 2010.
3. *Managing Performance Stress*, Routledge Press, 2006.

Chapter 7

STAYING WITH
THE PROGRAM:
NOT QUITTING

You wake up one morning, look out the window, and conclude that the sunshine and clear blue sky promise the dawning of a glorious day, perfect for doing the yard work you've been postponing for a while. You dress, grab some breakfast, and head to the tool shed. The weather inspires you; you feel great and know that being outside, bending, hauling, snipping, and digging will do you good. You'll work up a good appetite for lunch and feel terrific. Your motivation is unfettered and soaring. Off you go.

In this chapter we'll examine motivation for exercise and discuss ways to avoid quitting once you've begun.

Sometimes physical activities are done purely for fun and recreation, and fitness objectives are irrelevant or of secondary importance. On other occasions your exercise is a matter of obligation. You engage out of a sense of responsibility. The grass has to be mowed or the kitchen needs a fresh coat of paint. Duty calls. Your work is required. After all, it's your house. But you procrastinate. At the moment you don't feel like working. So you wait for the mood to strike. When you don't feel

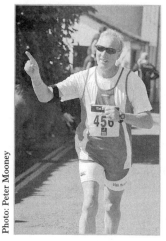

Photo: Peter Mooney

Motivation: we have all struggled with it, but some motivation must be cultivated and nurtured, just like muscle strength.

like cutting grass, you don't, and you grab paintbrushes and drop cloths only when the spirit moves you.

In the above scenario the need to do yard work was, of course, present. However, it was the pleasant weather that really inspired you. When your interests are centered upon self-improvement through exercise—when you truly appreciate the value of exercise, then the frequency and regularity of your engagement and the self-improvement goals you pursue take precedence over the color of the sky or amount of prevailing sunshine. Fair-weather exercising will yield but limited benefit. To get maximum pay-off you have to participate on a regular basis.

IN THE BEGINNING

In order to reduce the possibility of quitting, it helps to fully understand why you began your exercise program in the first place. Is it that you wish to be stronger, change your body's appearance, prevent muscular atrophy, or perhaps increase your flexibility?

Maybe you've read about recent scientific research that suggests a connection between memory and exercise. Lately, the popular press has been loaded with such revelations (see Chapter 4). Perhaps it's the social benefits available through membership in a health club or gym and desire to meet people and make new friends (also discussed in Chapter 4) that encourages you.

Whatever your motives are, it's a good bet that they differ from those of other exercisers. This is true not only because your mental, social, and physical needs and interests are probably different from many others in your own age group, but also because they are different from those in other age groups.

Undeniably, your teenage years are well behind you and you don't think, behave, or approach life the way adolescents do. So your motives for exercise are understandably not the same as those that inspire 15-, 16-, and 17-year-old kids.

Staying with the program and not quitting is perhaps the biggest challenge for exercisers of all ages, especially beginning exercisers. If you have not been involved in regular exercise for a long time, the necessary stick-to-itiveness may be difficult to achieve. The answer lies in the quality and strength of your *motivation*. (I'll define this term and discuss it shortly.)

Getting a good grip on your motivational level for almost any activity is essential to your staying power. The same is true of exercise. Some situations have higher levels of motivation than others. A scary diagnosis from your physician quickly cranks your motor, moves it out of idle, and throws it into overdrive. The doctor's words prompt a change in your behavior or lifestyle. In order to prevent worsening of a particular medical condition, you get on the ball and do it quickly. You don't procrastinate or proceed casually. You don't wait for nice weather. If your medical expert tells you to exercise you'd comply; or at least the chances are good that you would. If he insisted that you quit smoking, you'd hear him out and seriously consider his mandate—more earnestly and quickly than you would listen to that of a spouse or child. Doctors' opinions have credibility and they can initiate health behavior change and redirect your motivational dynamics.

I believe that it's fair to say that my portrayal of exercise as a clear and accessible route to well-being, contentment, and physiological health has been unfailing. Thematically, in every chapter I consistently hammer away in an effort to make a strong and rational case for exercise being universally essential to a high quality of existence. Some of you long ago came to understand the importance of regular physical activity and are already avid exercisers. Others are not there yet. To the uncommitted I say, "Get started now."

You need to be involved in some sort of physical activity on a regular basis. You need to change your health behavior, and you need to change it immediately. However, health behavior is not so easy to change. Those of you who have finally succeeded in disengaging from the powerful grip of tobacco dependency know of what I speak. It wasn't easy, was it? And for those of you who maintain that giving up tobacco wasn't so difficult, my bet is that some tumultuous experience impelled your attempt and eventual success—perhaps cardiovascular disease (heart attack) or emphysema, maybe a diagnosis of diabetes or perhaps a tumor found somewhere in your respiratory system. With the advent of these shocking revelations, you finally looked in the mirror and abruptly realized it was time to change. And this is how it went with my father.

Dad Did It

My father was a two-packs-a-day chain-smoker beginning in his teen years. When he was about 40 an X-ray revealed a spot on his lung that his physician declared to be "potentially troublesome." Fortunately, further tests revealed nothing of the sort and the collective sigh of relief exhaled by my family reverberated like a gale throughout the Bronx, New York City, where we lived. I vividly recall how he summoned my mother, brother, and me in to the parental bedroom, and with purpose and flair opened a drawer of his tall, upright dresser. From the drawer he lifted an aluminum cigarette case in which lay four of his Philip Morris cigarettes. He asked me to count them. "Four," I said. "Good," was his reply. "Now any time any of you want to count the number in this case again, you are welcome to come to my dresser and look. I'll never touch a cigarette again as long as I live."

And he didn't, all through the passing years. I was a boarder in my parents' home until my mid-20s and often visited his dresser drawer to check the contents of the aluminum case. Those four cigarettes lay there, untouched for almost 40 years. Dad kept his promise. He stopped smoking and did it cold turkey. To this day when I think of him I frequently recall this episode with a large measure of admiration. I'm sure that the spot on his lung and his contemplation of what it might have in store scared the pants off him. That's what it often takes to change deeply engrained and patterned health behavior.

INTENTIONAL CHANGE

J. O. Prochaska and his colleagues have written about five stages of change that occur. Over the years they have systematically applied it to problem behaviors such as overeating, smoking, drinking, weight control, condom use for HIV protection, and drug abuse. According to their Transtheoretical Model (fancy name, but not all that complicated to understand) my father really didn't cut loose from his tobacco habit in one fell swoop. He actually did it over time after considerable emotional and cognitive involvement.

Let's have a look at this model in terms of our interest in failure to exercise on a regular basis. I'm herewith designating this failure a problem behavior and adding it to the list of Prochaska's behaviors cited above. I'm saying that not exercising regularly or not sustaining the activity program over time constitutes a tangible and acute health problem.

The Transtheoretical Model is a template or pattern for intentional change—change that at some level of awareness a person really wants to make. The model suggests that an individual confronts his or her admitted health-related problem (smoking, etc.) and eventually takes the bull by the horns. A model is an illustration or representation of something that is proposed in theory. A model airplane represents or describes a much larger machine that actually flies. The Transtheoretical Model explains how meaningful behavior change occurs over time. Emotions and thoughts are involved at first when the individual considers the benefits and disadvantages of change (all the issues we've been talking about in the previous six chapters).

In stage one of the model, the *precontemplation stage*, the intention to take action within the foreseeable future (the next six months) is not present. The individual is uninformed or inadequately informed about the consequences of their problem behavior (not exercising). If you have digested the materials presented in the preceding six chapters you should not fall into this category. You should be well informed about the pitfalls of not exercising. Sometimes someone who has previously tried to change a spotlighted behavior but has failed is said to be in this stage.

In stage two, the *contemplation stage*, the intention to change (within the next six months) is expressed. Those in this stage have considered both pros and cons of changing their behavior and declare a desire for change. But as they think about advantages and disadvantages (what's involved in seeking the change) they may become confused, overly deliberative, and consequently, stage stuck. They just continue to mull over both sides of the coin and despite their expression of desire for change, are mired in inaction.

In stage three, the *preparation stage*, the intention to change is present, but in addition some significant action has taken place. A chat about exercise with a physician has occurred, so has signing up at a health club. Acquisition of and reading this book is another example of significant action. The person in this stage of the model is ripe for change.

The fourth stage of the Transtheoretical Model is the stage of *action*, wherein observable behavior directly related to the target actually occurs. The individual begins attending the health club or dance class. She becomes an exerciser and demonstrates an effort to avoid returning to the prior behavior (not exercising) that required change in the first place.

In the fifth and final stage, *maintenance*, the person is not highly tempted to fall off the wagon (relapse) and shows more and more confidence in the ability to sustain the changed behavior.

So, where are you now? In what stage of behavior change are you located? If you are in stages one through four, move forward. Try to transition into stage five of the Transtheoretical Model and become a regular exerciser.

MOTIVATION: THE WHY AND DIRECTION OF BEHAVIOR

Think of *motivation* as *the force that propels your behavior in a certain direction*. Think of it as *the energy that pushes you to do something, or not do something*. Your doctor's admonishment and prognosis in the above example activated behavior. Your degree of motivation is specific to each situation in which you are involved. Your energy for attending a baseball game may be greater than it is for sitting through an opera performance. Or the reverse may be true. Your level of energy for going shopping for new living room furniture may be higher than it is for doing laundry.

In order to stay with your exercise program you must be in touch with what motivates you. Talk to yourself. Ask yourself questions about your motivation. "Why have I commited to regular exercise? For vanity or health? Do I really believe that participating in an exercise regimen will result in positive change? Can I really do this? Will I really do this?" Your internal dialogue can shape and strengthen it. Mull these questions over in order to gain insight into the why of your decision. This is yet another way to approach the term motivation. Motivation can also be understood as *the why of behavior*.

The Energizer Bunny™ you've seen in battery commercials on television and in magazines, just keeps going, going, going, and going. He's the little guy you want to emulate when embarking upon an exercise program. But first you must have insight into the nature and degree of your motivation. And you must also be as realistic as possible when setting your exercise goals. I can't emphasize this enough. If you are overly ambitious, the probability of quitting increases and quitting is an undesirable agenda item. Here's your guiding concept: *In order to derive anticipated benefit from your exercise program, you must stick with it.*

Despite the fact that some short-term advantages may result from even a single bout of exercise, you should strive for long-term involvement and withdraw only when legitimate reasons intervene. Admirable as it may be to begin exercising upon advice from your physician, it's better if you arrive at the decision to do so on your own. When you do, what sets you off is called *intrinsic* or *internal motivation*. The physician who pushes you to begin an exercise program would be considered an *external* or *extrinsic motivator*. Both are valuable, but motivation that comes from within is more effective.

OF MICE AND MEN

Some evidence from animal studies suggests that motivation for exercise might even be related to hereditary factors. This being the case, it may not be your doctor, spouse, or children who inspire your entry into exercise. It may be your genes that contribute influentially to your motivation for exercise. I've previously commented about studies that have used mice as subjects and how some findings have prompted research into various exercise-related phenomena in humans.

Here are some additional findings:

1. Hereditary factors transmitted from parent mouse offspring seem to inspire a tendency toward physical activity.[1]

2. Digit length (fingers) in white mice seems to correlate with desire to exercise. Those rodents with long digits have a stronger desire to exercise than those with shorter fingers.[2]

So you're smirking and thinking, "What has this got to do with me? I'm not a rodent." Well, scientists are now considering a possible link between a number of personality traits (including a propensity for rigorous physical activity) and length of ring finger in humans. Wow! Please don't disparage results from rodent research. Despite the multitude of superficial differences between mice and humans, many of the systems and physiological mechanisms are very similar. We continue to learn a lot about the ways in which we behave, learn, and think from studies that employ these little animals.

How to Achieve and Sustain High Levels of Motivation

Your motivation for just about any activity or behavior may very well be influenced by your personality (I touched upon this in Chapter 6). And personality, in turn, may have genetic links. This explains why some of us find it easier to be motivated for almost anything than others we know. Whether or not you are endowed with *motivational genes*, the choice to exercise is basically yours. Here are some suggestions that should help you develop and sustain high levels of motivation for exercise.

1. *Be sure to establish realistic exercise goals.* (More about this in Chapter 8.) Attend to the signals provided by your body about fatigue and discomfort. Don't overdo it. And perhaps

most important of all, don't permit exercise to be disagreeable. Discomfort during or after exercise will undermine motivation to maintain your program.

Let common sense be your guide. Back off when your body tells you to. You've been around a long time and have had many conversations with your body. Listen to the messages and be prepared to retreat. This business of *no pain, no gain* is sheer nonsense, and in my opinion, baseless even for elite or professional athletes. You don't have to be in pain to progress in your exercise program.

2. *Select a location for your exercise that is easily accessible.* If you have to solve logistical problems in order to get to your exercise venue your motivation level will take a hit. Your focus will shift from the pleasure of exercise and its beneficial outcomes to dealing with driving or transportation hassles. Consider how far you must travel to get to the tennis court and whether you'll be able to find a partner every time you wish to play.

I've known people who selected exercise clubs or gyms solely on the basis of membership fee. Because one was cheaper than others they opted for one while overlooking the amount of travel time and gas required to make the trip. These turned out to be detriments to their motivation, and consequently, they quit.

3. *Determine the kind of physical environment that is satisfying and arrange to do your exercise there.* For instance, do you enjoy solitude? Are you content to be alone? Does the beauty and wonder of nature excite and gratify you? Are you attracted to flowers, plants, scurrying animals, and chirping birds? If you are, then build such elements into your exercise environment. Try to exercise where you'll experience sights, sounds, and events that provide pleasure.

Perhaps you are you the kind of person who prefers to be in the company of others and likes to chat with friends while doing things? If so, take such interests into account when planning your program. Where you exercise is an important element of your motivation for physical activity. Make an effort to ensure exercise satisfaction by carefully selecting an environment that is pleasing. If a gym is where you intend to exercise, find out when the noise level and number of exercisers are compatible with your needs and tolerance levels. Certain times of the day accommodate very large crowds and make exercise venues noisy.

The important thing is to be aware of your preferences and decide accordingly. Your exercise need not occur in a gym, athletic field, or even outdoors. Your preference—and a most legitimate one at that—may be for your own home, rec room, basement, or yard. Think about location and decide based on what's best for you.

4. *Pay attention to the weather when planning your exercise program.* Prevailing weather conditions should be factored into your activity choices if you want to sustain high motivational levels. Are you comfortable doing yard work in summer heat or shoveling snow in winter frost? Does rain or high humidity bother you to the extent that you'd call off walking or cycling? If your answers to these questions reveal a preference for a particular climate, it's likely that your motivational level for physical activity will diminish if weather that you dislike prevails.

What happens if you decide that shoveling snow daily will be your exercise during the winter months? You plan to kill two birds with one stone; you'll accomplish something practical, and in one swoop also satisfy your need for daily exercise. But can you rely on consistent and adequate snowfall where you live so as to satisfy your plan and sustain a high level of motivation?

In this case, an alternate plan would be a good idea. Back up your snow-shoveling strategy with something indoors, just in case. This way when the weather doesn't cooperate, you'll still be motivated to exercise. Along these lines, consider the best time of day for participation in your program of physical activity. An unwise choice will certainly interfere with attempts to remain motivated.

I live in Florida where the heat and humidity are substan-

tial during the late spring, summer, and early fall. Walking
and jogging and, for that matter, most outdoor activities are
stressful and uncomfortable if not done in the early morning
or late evening hours. I know this and plan my exercise activities accordingly. I take care of daily exercise in early morning when the air is cool and the traffic not as formidable.

5. *Give some thought to the frequency of your exercise.* Will you
   participate every day or a few times a week? And what is the
   basis for your decision? Unless you are preparing for competition and seek very high degrees of fitness, three times a
   week should be sufficient. *Approximately* 20 to 30 minutes of
   aerobic activity should be enough.

   And your activity program should be varied: some aerobic
   work, some flexibility training, and some strength-building
   activity. Balance is the keynote; not too much of any one kind
   of activity is best. All of the preceding components of your
   exercise program need not be included on a daily basis. You
   can walk, jog, or cycle every other day and concentrate on
   strength activities in between. But it's a good idea to stretch
   every day. I'll have more to say about this in Chapter 8,
   when I address avoiding exercise injury.

   A friend of mine with an interest in shedding some weight
   now exercises at the gym during lunch hour. His reason?
   Here's his answer: "This way I skip lunch, save calories and
   money, and get to sleep in a little longer in the morning, my
   previous time for exercise." Without commenting upon the
   advisability of missing the noon meal, I simply offer this
   time switch as an illustration of a motivational dynamic. It
   exemplifies my point about individual needs and interests.

WHAT TO WEAR DURING EXERCISE

Clothes may make the man, but do they also make the exerciser? This question has a little more substance to it than meets
the eye. Inappropriate selection of exercise apparel can account
for being uncomfortable to the extent that exercise is cut short.
If you are too warm or too cold, you'll quit earlier than
planned.

Aging is often accompanied by altered sensitivities to environmental temperatures. Kids can run around outdoors in t-shirts on the coolest of days, while older exercisers may require a covering of some sort. So keep something handy in case the weather changes. Throw a sweater or comfortable body cover in your gym bag or car trunk. A windbreaker or sweatshirt can always be removed and wrapped around your waist if you are too warm during exercise.

And it's a good idea to keep the body's large skeletal muscles warm at the outset of your workout. Warm muscles generally function more efficiently than cold ones. That's one reason why athletes warm up before competition. Prior to leaving the house, check the temperature outside and consider the day's forecast. Avoid exercising vigorously out of doors when the temperature exceeds 80° F. Even highly trained younger exercisers are cautioned by the American College of Sports Medicine against taking an outside workout when the thermometer reaches this point.

And speaking about what to wear in conjunction with motivation, consider this: If you are a morning exerciser lay out your stuff near your bed before you retire. This will enable visual contact with your sneakers, gym bag, warm-up suit, cap, or whatever, as soon as you throw your legs over the edge of the bed. You'll be reminded of your commitment first thing. Do the same with your gardening outfit or cycling clothes. (Always wear a helmet when riding and be certain that it fits properly and covers as much of your head as possible.) This way, before you hit the bathroom or kitchen you'll have already taken an important first step.

Protection of the body is another reason for making appropriate choices about exercise apparel. Your exercise routine may require that you come in contact with abrasive surfaces. When ice-skating or roller-blading, you are likely to take an occasional tumble irrespective of your level of competence. Even the most fit and skillful exercisers have a mishap now and then. Elbow, hand, and knee coverings are therefore a good idea.

Sun block is a must for all activities out of doors, and it's wise to have head covering as well. Remember, not all outdoor physical activity involves running or moving the body rapidly through space. Gardening, croquet, and golf also require appropriate head and body covering in addition to sun block. Sunglasses should be worn when exercising out of doors. As we age, vulnerability to eye conditions such as macular degeneration and cataracts increases. Sunglasses with adequate ultraviolet sunray protection may reduce the cause or progression of such conditions.

Yet another dimension of exercise attire is appearance—how you believe others see you. Recall that I previously mentioned the social objectives of exercise. I indicated that meeting people and establishing new relationships are legitimate motivations for beginning and maintaining an exercise program. Today, exercise apparel follows fashion and is varied and popular. No longer are exercisers satisfied with old t-shirts and worn tennis shoes. Within almost any sport or exercise category, attractive options are available for specialized attire.

You can find footwear especially designed for everything from badminton to volleyball. And many people purchase and dress in exercise outfits for casual wear simply to be in vogue. Think for a moment of the people you know of any age who wear running shoes, baseball caps, and warm-up suits for nonexercise activities. So why not look spiffy when exercising?

You'll probably be under the watchful eyes of friends or potential friends while at the tennis court, swimming pool, and gym or while square dancing at the senior center. Treat yourself to a nice outfit; you'll feel good about yourself and about exercise. But be careful to select style, color, and size that do your body justice. Your appearance should reflect an attractive older person secure in his or her *body image*, a man or woman not in competition with teenagers or popular movie actors or actresses.

BODY IMAGE

Body image is the view you hold of your physical self. That is, your view of your body and its parts. It also reflects your feelings (no one else's) about the way in which your body functions. Comments such as "I'm clumsy," "I'm a fast walker," or

"I'm very tall" are indicative of your body image. And your body view is related to the way in which you picture your entire self, better known as the *self-concept*. The self-concept is a critical part of your psychology. It affects your behavior, your attitudes about the world in which you function, and the extent to which you pursue and achieve established goals.

Flattering comments from fellow exercisers as to your appearance not only help shape your body image and self-concept, but also assist in strengthening your motivation for exercise. Exercise attire is a link between appearance and self-concept. When you like the way you look, your body view is strengthened. A strong body image contributes to a well-developed self-concept. People with well-developed and healthy concepts of self are comfortable with themselves. They are secure in their identity and confident in their interactions with others.

Exercise clothing need not be skimpy or revealing. Both good taste and personal budgetary considerations should dictate what you purchase and wear. But by all means, give attention to your appearance. Other exercisers will. Believe it or not, what an exercise leader wears also influences perceptions of class members about the value and effectiveness of what transpires in class.

In a study we conducted at my university (Steve Wininger's doctoral dissertation), we learned that the way members of an aerobic dance class evaluated their instructor had to do with what she was wearing. If members of the class liked the leader's costume or thought she looked nice, they tended to judge the value of the class very favorably in comparison to classes led by instructors whose attire was not approved. We found something similar with regard to the music played during class. If participants liked the music, their evaluations of the class were favorable. If the music didn't appeal to them the ratings were considerably lower.

Have you noticed that those leaving an exercise class or gym often comment upon the experience in terms of the music that might have been playing? "I didn't enjoy the class because the music was too loud" or "I hate rap." "Why couldn't he have played something more to my liking?"

MUSIC

Music can have an *ergogenic* effect upon your motivation during exercise. By this I mean that it can be inspiring, stimulating, and effort enhancing. Pep bands and marching units at football and basketball games are used strategically to arouse fans as well as athletes. As suggested in Chapter 6, in activities that require a good deal of concentration, this arousal may be undesirable. Nonetheless, in many exercise activities, including yard work, jogging, walking, and weight lifting, music can have a desirable impact on your involvement. It's worth a try.

While working in the yard next time, turn on the radio and listen to music you like. If you are exposed to a neighbor's music that you find disagreeable, the opposite effect may kick in. But on the other hand, if the activity requires strength or heavy lifting, annoying music might conceivably be helpful. The music's disagreeability might actually activate you and result in a better performance. It's probably not a good idea to listen to

---

AN INTERESTING LITTLE TIDBIT:
"SENIOR DANCE TEAMS SCORE ON NBA COURTS"
(AARP Bulletin, October 2010, Vol. 51, No. 8.)

Senior dance squads that perform at NBA games have been sprouting up in recent years, proving that showmanship isn't just for the young. About a dozen dance teams shimmy to pop and hip-hop beats at halftime for fired-up basketball fans.

"Who would think we'd be doing this when we retire?" asks Freya Sherman, 65, of the Villages, Florida. She and her husband, Gerry, 67, dance with the Orlando Magic's Silver Stars. La Verna Rodriguez, 82, of North Phoenix, Arizona, entertains with the Phoenix Suns' Golden Grannies. "Just because you're old doesn't mean you have to sit around and do nothing," she says. Competition is stiff. Between 50 and 100 participants typically try out for the Chicago Bulls' Swinging Seniors. Last year, 14 made the team. Director Cathy Core marvels at the dancers' hard work and enthusiasm. "You expect certain things, and they deliver."

music while playing tennis or golf because the demands upon your attention and the need to focus on court events would hamper your ability to appreciate the music.

Many walkers use headphones plugged into devices that provide music. Unfortunately, this may interfere with the safety of the walk in that awareness of traffic and other important things transpiring in the environment is compromised. So be careful, but realize that music and exercise may make very good partners. If you are not a music fan, perhaps a short story or informative lecture might fill the bill, particularly when doing exercise that doesn't require a good deal of high-level thinking or problem solving.

MODELING: MOTIVATION THROUGH OBSERVING OTHER EXERCISERS

When your inspiration for almost any kind of behavior or activity depends on what others are doing or how others may look, when you admire people to the extent that you wish to appear like them and then copy their behavior, attitude, or emotional expressions, the process involved is known as *modeling*. Even behavior observed in others that involves self-control (important in weight regulation) can be contagious. This can also happen with exercise.

The impact of modeling upon your motivation for exercise can be very strong, but it really depends upon the type of model you are emulating. If the object of your modeling is someone who is close to you in physical characteristics and abilities, then the process is empowered. If you are 80 years of age and your model is a professional athlete of 20, modeling can get you into trouble. You'll try to replicate the model's behavior to your detriment and it's very likely that you'll injure yourself. But if you choose a model prudently and realistically, your motivation for exercise should be enhanced.

The most effective kinds of models are those people who have much in common with you. The closer you are in as many characteristics as possible to the person whose behavior you intend to emulate, the more effective the process will be. So for example, when observing someone of similar age, gender, family situation, and socioeconomic status, who is engaged happily and profitably in exercise, chances are good that you'll model this behavior advantageously. When you recognize significant distinctions between yourself and someone else—say for instance, he or she is much younger, thinner, or not married (and you are)—then the probability of using his or her behavior (in this case, exercise) as an effective model is marginal.

All of us absorb a lot from watching others, including inspiration to exercise. But modeling can also have a down side. That's why parents disapprove of their kids playing with certain children who they feel will exert undesirable influences. Or why you prefer not to socialize with an acquaintance because you notice that when in his company your own behavior tends to be as unpleasant as his. For reasons you don't exactly understand you seem to act like him, and you really don't care to be that way.

You can also pick up negative attitudes about exercise from others through modeling. Those who disdain what they consider to be unnecessary physical activity but who have a number of other things in common with you and are similar to you in many respects and for whom you have a high regard may reduce your enthusiasm for exercise. Because you like them or value your association with them, they have an impact upon your thinking.

In a similar vein, their reluctance to exercise might unfortunately give you reason to reflect upon your plans to begin a walking or yoga program. So it's a two-way street. When it comes to motivation, modeling can influence you positively or negatively. One interesting observation that recently came to my attention fits in nicely here. When exercisers—in this case, members of a rowing team—trained together, they were able to tolerate twice as much pain as measured on a pain tolerance test administered after the workout. Evidently, working together (perhaps modeling?) has an impact on pain tolerance.

☞ WHAT YOU'VE LEARNED IN THIS CHAPTER

Motivation for exercise was this chapter's primary focus. You
were encouraged to think of motivation as the energy behind
everything you do, as well as the reason or reasons you have
behaved in certain ways. With regard to exercise and its benefits, maintaining high levels of enthusiasm for the program is
absolutely essential and dropping out interferes with achievement of your health and fitness objectives. An essential part of
keeping your motivation high is understanding why you began
exercising in the first place. This insight will both reduce the
likelihood of quitting and strengthen your determination to
continue.

A five-stage model—the Transtheoretical Model—was presented in order to point out that changing a health behavior
takes time.

A number of suggestions for keeping motivation strong and
intact were provided in the chapter. Setting realistic exercise
goals and considering the location of your exercise place, as
well as its distance from where you live or work, contribute to
motivation. An irritating exercise environment or one that involves stressful travel can undermine your resolve.

Exercise clothing can stimulate enthusiasm for participation.
Dress nicely, comfortably, and in a fashion that suits your appearance. Factor into your exercise choices the weather, the
time of day in which you are likely to participate, and the
probability of your being able to sustain your program as seasons change. Certain forms of physical activity require being
out of doors. Therefore, in order to maintain regular participation, take into account seasonal climate shifts when planning
your program.

Music that you enjoy can provide comfort that will make exercise more attractive. Not all exercise venues are gyms or spas.
Sometimes people exercise in their bedrooms, yards, or neighborhoods. Arrange to listen to enjoyable or stimulating music
in order to maintain high motivational levels.

One other factor that influences your motivation for exercise is modeling, or identifying with persons you know and admire. A desire to be like them or look like them (or not look like them) can increase your drive to exercise regularly.

FOOD FOR THOUGHT

1. Try to identify reasons for your deciding to bring regular exercise into your life. Is it your physician who is providing the motivation? Are you responding to encouragement from a friend or highly regarded relative? Are you dissatisfied with your appearance and wish to lose weight or reconfigure your body contours? Examine your motives and determine if your reasons are legitimate, reasonable, and sustainable.

2. Occasionally assess your progress toward exercise goals. Are you losing or putting on weight? (Either can be an appropriate goal.) Also assess your attitudes about exercise on a periodic basis. Are you really enjoying what you are doing? Try to determine the reason underlying your answer to this question. Why are you (or are you not) deriving satisfaction from exercise? Use these answers as a basis for modifying or continuing your program and its elements.

3. Construct a plan to put into effect when and if your motivation weakens. Perhaps what you are doing is too heavily oriented toward strength training. Or perhaps the aerobic component is too challenging for you and depriving you of the required satisfaction and enjoyment of participation. Perhaps the model you are emulating is inappropriate even though you are of comparable age and background.

Making Choices

Good choices are the building blocks for high levels of motivation. To stay with your program after having initiated it, be certain you've clarified the needs underlying your decision to embark upon an exercise program. Assess the importance of beginning your program to the various aspects of your life (social, health fitness, and so on). Have a look at your readiness to begin. What is your degree of physical ability? Are you emotionally prepared to start? Is this a good time?

Making the Commitment

FOUR SIMPLE QUESTIONS

The following questions should help you focus upon important exercise–motivational issues. Contemplate each one carefully before responding.

1. At this time a regular program of exercise would be . . .
   a. not important or not good for me.
   b. very important and good for me.

2. How much exercise would be appropriate for me at this time?
   a. three times a week for about 30 minutes
   b. four times a week for about 30 minutes
   c. three times a week for more than 30 minutes
   d. four times a week for more than 30 minutes

3. What's my best choice for an activity? Why?

4. Am I ready?

Endnotes

1. Garland et al., 2010.
2. Manning & Taylor, 2001.
3. Cohen, Ejsmond-Frey, Knight, & Dunbar, 2010.

Chapter 8

SETTING EXERCISE GOALS: ESTABLISHING THE PHYSICAL ACTIVITY PLAN

Have a plan for each and every exercise session. Pre-
determine what you want to accomplish and base
your decision upon how you perceive personal health
and fitness. Understand exactly what you are capable of achieving, how much time you have at your
disposal, and which element or elements of your fitness require change. Be sure that any advice you
have received, no matter what the source, is the very
best you can find.

To effectively improve your mental and physical health, regulate your body weight, and manage stress and anxiety through exercise, it must be done properly. By *properly* I mean that it is to be done insightfully, safely, sensibly, correctly, and regularly. Enthusiasm and commitment are also vital ingredients and byproducts of a high level of motivation (see Chapter 7), but alone they are insufficient. All components must be incorporated because each contributes to your readiness to begin your activity program. You also need a detailed plan in which desired outcomes are identified and anticipated challenges envisioned and clearly stated. All of these requirements

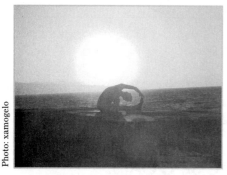

Photo: xamogelo

Just as we set goals in our daily life, from sunrise to sunset, setting exercise goals are fundamental to seeing progress. We must always see what lies ahead.

are part and parcel of a process known as *goal setting*, which is precisely the focus of this chapter.

In sport a goal is a tally, a point, an achievement. It's something recorded on the scoreboard; it's a piece of data, a statistic that indicates what is ahead. At the end of the contest, if the total number of goals earned by a team in lacrosse, soccer, water polo, football, or hockey is greater than the opponent has scored, victory accrues. Simply stated—more goals equates with winning. That's what the word *goal* means in sport. In the context of this chapter, it means something else.

When I refer to exercise goals here I have in mind an eye to the future, rather than something accomplished in the recent past. I'm talking about what you intend to accomplish rather than what you or your team has just achieved. Think of exercise goals as outcomes that lead to some sort of important and desired change. Each goal you set is akin to an agenda item.

However, the sequence in which they are to be achieved must be carefully planned. If itemized realistically and sequenced correctly and logically, your exercise goals stand a good chance of being realized. The ultimate result is a change in your behavior, not just any behavior but one that is targeted by no one else but you. In this case it's a modification in various elements of physical fitness, well-being, and health (see Chapter 2).

When you establish meaningful exercise or fitness goals, pursue, and eventually accomplish them, you strengthen your motivation for further physical activity because you see improvement and positive change. Each successfully accomplished goal reinforces your journey toward improved health and fitness. Each goal achieved provides impetus for continuing in what you now perceive to be the correct direction. You realize this— sense that you are doing the right thing and are encouraged to continue. You become more and more secure that your quest will eventually be completely successful.

Goal setting is certainly not unique to exercise. Its use is widespread in the worlds of business, organizational leadership, and behavior change in so many other areas. But its applications in what is known as *exercise psychology* have yielded excellent results.

GOAL SETTING: GETTING STARTED

The following seven steps compose a goal-setting pathway. They are presented in question format. As you respond and follow the recommendations associated with each one you'll be moving forward resolutely, moving toward behavior change.

Step 1: Where do you want to be? What's your fitness target?
Consider what preferred fitness end-point you seek. Think about what you really want to be like, to look like, to feel like. What kind of physical performances do you wish to ultimately achieve? What is important that you desire to accomplish physically and cannot do presently or can do only with difficulty?

When others, particularly those whose assessments you care about, see you and observe your movements and physical function, how do you wish them to evaluate you? What images do you hold about your physical appearance? Upon what criteria are these images predicated?

Honest answers to these questions are the foundation of effective goal setting. But this important self-assessment should not be exclusively focused on external features, such as your waist size or muscular development. A significant piece of your envisioned model should also relate to your internal functions, operations that are ongoing inside your body that are not ostensible, internal activities that are reflective of your health, well-being, and fitness.

You've seen photos that depict idealized human lung and heart tissue, and illustrations of blood vessels, ligaments, tendons, and bones. They adorn the walls of your physician's little examining rooms in which you sit forever and ever, awaiting his or her entry. You sit patiently on the examining table and eventually your attention gravitates to the charts and posters on the wall.

Somewhere along the line, as you've developed into an aware older individual, you've acquired mental pictures that portray healthy and properly functioning vital organs and systems. You have an idea what they should look like. If you don't, pay closer attention to the television commercials that advertise various medications and chemical remedies; they are often accompanied by animated representations of your internal organic anatomies and operations. Or check available magazines that include advertisements for pills, tablets, liquids, and lotions. From such sources formulate an idea of what you aspire to be like and look like internally.

And speaking of television, be wary of the multitude of so-called infomercials that peddle magical machines and dietary supplements designed to "flatten your stomach," "burn calories without exercise," or "convert fat to muscle." First of all, your stomach is an internal organ like your pancreas or liver. You don't access or strengthen it by doing sit-ups or any other kind of abdominal workout on any kind of device. And with regard to burning calories without doing exercise— well, you are always using calories, even during rest or sleep. But you burn more during physical activity.

Alas, there's no free lunch (review parts of Chapter 3). If you want to increase the number of calories you utilize during a 24-hour period, increasing your physical activity will help. Lastly, body tissue is body tissue. You can't convert nerve cells to bone cells, blood cells to muscle cells, or fat to muscle. Period. Many of these claims are truly without scientific validity, despite their advocates' claims to the contrary.

Step 2: How realistic are the body images you've constructed? You're older but you don't have one foot in the grave. You're also not 15 or 20 anymore. Truth be told, you can no longer look or even feel like a 20-year-old. If you haven't yet accepted this, please do so now. The idea is to look and feel like an attractive Boomer man or woman. That's what I mean by being honest in constructing your body portrait.

Are the criteria you've established and the visions and aspirations revealed through your self-analyses, authentic? Have you really been straightforward in your assessments? Or have you envisioned what is perhaps a desirable, culturally sanctioned but realistically unattainable person? Run a reality check. Be assured that you've been fair to yourself. Return to Step 1 and answer the same questions again.

Step 3: Are you ready to begin an exercise program? Evaluate your readiness to begin a regular program of physical activity, one specifically designed to satisfy your authentic self-images. What's your level of psychological preparedness to proceed with this quest? (See Chapter 7.) Many exercisers are motivated purely by recreational interests. This is fine, even commendable. A sound fitness program may certainly include a hefty recreational component. But are you ready to move forward with a fitness training regimen? Mind you, *fitness* is a primary concern in this book.

On a scale of 1 to 10, where is your readiness located? (I'm spinning off of what we discussed in Chapter 7, namely the Transtheoretical Model by Prochaska and colleagues.)

- Give yourself a 1 if your reply is something like this: "Regular exercise is absolutely out of the question for me, at least right now. I'm not at all interested."

- Score a 2 or 3 if your answer is a version of this: "On occasion I consider starting a program of fitness training—but I don't think I'm very serious about it."

- Assign a 4 or 5 if you respond with something like this: "I believe I'm beyond mere thinking occasionally about exercise. Lately I've been giving serious thought to doing something about my fitness, but I'm not quite ready to take action."

- Your score would be about 6 if your attitude is, "I'd begin if I had someone to join me or if I had available leadership that would give me a shove."

- An answer like this would deserve a 7: "I think I'm ready, but perhaps next month would be a better time to get started than this week. I've got too many things on my to-do list."

- Your score would be 8 or 9 if you responded in the following fashion: "You know, maybe I'm really ready. Perhaps I'll speak this week with some people who know about exercise and get some advice, ask them what they do, and where they do it."

- If you feel that you're absolutely raring to go and can't wait to get started, you should award yourself a 10, especially if your statement was anything like this: "I regret having put it off for so long. I should have begun a long time ago."

This book should be helpful no matter your location on the scale. The first four chapters provide insight into the benefits of exercise, particularly for readers over the age of sixty. If necessary, re-read these chapters, or at least read the summary sections again. See if your self-assigned position on the readiness scale changes.

You are now in the midst of Chapter 8, which suggests a fairly keen interest in exercise. You wouldn't have read this far if you weren't at least moderately interested. You've learned about various exercise issues and how and why exercise is vital to your health and well-being. You should be at about level 8 or 9—nothing less. You know about the psychological and physiological benefits of exercise, about avoidance of exercise injury, and about nutritional considerations that accompany a program of physical fitness. My hunch is that you are probably ready.

Step 4: When should you exercise? When you set goals, you should give attention to this issue.

Think about your personal patterns of daily commitments. Consider your standing appointments, ones that are constant and rigid. For instance, perhaps you help out with grandchildren by delivering them to school or picking them up; maybe you meet regularly with the guys or women for coffee at 9 each morning; possibly you play cards with friends every Wednesday at 3 p.m. or volunteer at the local hospital at noon twice a week in order to relieve employees for their lunch break. Whatever the case, be cognizant of these scheduled and valued events.

Next, identify a time block that is free. Set aside about an hour. You can get by with a little less, but if you factor in preparation time (gathering and putting on appropriate clothing or equipment), the exercise itself, and putting away equipment and showering afterwards, you'll need at least an hour, or close to it. This does not include time necessary for travel to the exercise venue.

In making decisions about when to exercise, bear in mind a number of critical factors. Is your exercise of choice to be conducted out of doors or indoors? If you intend to satisfy your exercise interests by gardening or walking out of doors, you'll have to contend with varying weather conditions. Seasonal changes may bring cold or elevated heat and humidity. Identify your likes and dislikes in terms of climate. Do you enjoy a nip in the air or do you prefer to stay indoors during the cooler seasons? Think about such things lest you make an unsupportable commitment as you respond to the vagaries of weather and fluctuating temperatures. Or have contingency plans.

Let's say you've decided to establish a walking program, and you reside in the northeast part of the United States. Consider indoor walking facilities that might be at your disposal during winter's inclement weather. An indoor mall or local gymnasium with a track could be established as backup facilities. But this requires planning. Be sure these places are available at the hour you wish to exercise. Determine whether or not you are welcome and whether a fee is required.

Give thought to your *circadian rhythms*. Here I refer to the changes in your biochemical and organic function occurring rhythmically during a 24-hour period. These cyclical patterns are individually set; that is, they are idiosyncratic or person specific. They account for some of us being morning persons while others have a marked preference for almost any type of activity—intellectual or physical—later in the day.

A former colleague of mine knew that the best time for him to concentrate on his professional writing was after dinner in the evening, at about 9 p.m. This was when he was most productive as a scholar, when he could think, write, and analyze without fatigue or distraction. Not so for me.

I have known myself to be a morning person for a long, long time, since I was a high school student. When studying for exams and later on, doing my professional writing, I've always been much better off attacking my work early in the day. That's also when I do my exercise. I'm at the gym or track by 5:30 a.m. After supper, I can't think straight. I get sleepy. I'm dislodged from my preferred and productive slip stream. So I restrict my activities to light reading, a crossword puzzle, or watching some television. This kind of arrangement suits me.

However, it may not be the best way for you to do things. If you are still in the work force, then career obligations will influence your chosen time for programmed physical activity. You have little choice but to do your exercise before, after, or perhaps during a lunch break. No scheduling choices are right or wrong for everyone, just arrangements that are right or wrong for you. If you overlook your circadian rhythms when planning your program, you may conceivably sacrifice potential motivation and enthusiasm for exercise (see Chapter 7).

Step 5: Are your exercise goals as highly specific as possible? In setting exercise goals it is essential at the outset that the goals be specific. Goals that are too broadly stated will not only be unhelpful, but they can undermine your well-intentioned efforts. Consider the following examples. One exemplifies a weak or inappropriate goal-setting attempt because it is not specific, and the other portrays a properly stated goal.

1. "I want to be stronger." This goal is too general. It's lacking in specificity. It doesn't inform the exerciser precisely what is to be accomplished.

2. "At the end of next month my goal is to demonstrate an increase in five pounds of muscular strength in both left and right biceps muscles." This statement is pointed, specific, and helpful in that it lays out very clearly what the exerciser seeks to accomplish in a particular time frame.

Here's another example of a good and not so good exercise goal.

1. "I want to be able to walk faster." (not good)

2. "My goal is to walk a mile in less than 18 minutes by the end of June." (good)

When your goal or goals have been articulated, publish them. Post them prominently, somewhere that indicates by their location their importance, somewhere they are readily viewable by you. The refrigerator door or bathroom mirror are excellent places, if no one else in the house objects. Goal publication serves as a reminder that you've made a commitment, that you are serious about modifying your fitness status.

The above examples use muscular strength and walking-speed to make a point about goal specificity. But don't forget what was emphasized in Chapters 1 and 4—not everyone need select a regimen of calisthenics, weight training, jogging, or walking as their exercise of choice. As I've repeatedly explained, you should choose the form of physical activity that is best for you, considering your interests, health, and current fitness level. But you've got to do something. You've got to be active physically. And one important ingredient in constructing your exercise plan is the establishment of realistic goals.

Step 6: Are your goals short as well as long term?
Not all goals are aimed at the distant future. Your goal setting should have both short- and long-term targets. Each workout session (daily or every other day or three times a week, whatever the case) requires a set of goals. All of the examples provided in Step 5 are of the long-term kind; however, short-termers should also be part of your thinking and planning. For instance: "Tomorrow, when I pull weeds in the garden, I plan to stay on my knees for 10 more minutes than I was able to two weeks ago." Or, "In today's pool workout, I intend to swim at least one more lap doing crawl stroke and one less lap doing breast stroke before completing my 200 yards."

(Lest I forget, let me here recommend a wonderful book for those of you who are or who intend to be swimmers. It's extremely comprehensive in its approach to all aspects of swimming and I believe that it will be very helpful: *Swimming for Total Fitness—A Progressive Aerobic Program*, by Jane Katz. Dr. Katz is a champion Masters Swimmer and a distinguished member of the Boomer and beyond generation.)

These (above) short-term goals express exercise objectives to be accomplished in the immediate future (tomorrow or today), in contrast to others that are set in the distant future (next month, by the end of June, etc.).

Step 7: Are your goals realistic and attainable?
Young children often announce desired performance targets that are completely fanciful. As you listen to a child describe anticipated exercise accomplishments, your wealth of past experiences dictates that the little girl or boy is way off base. You know that the child is expressing nothing more than wishful thinking, and you are confident that the child's goals will not be fulfilled. Perhaps you smile, or if you are intent

upon being a good advisor, teacher, parent, or grandparent, you might discretely offer a suggestion or two with the hope that the child modifies his or her goals. Adults are also not immune to proclaiming pie-in-the-sky aspirations. Fortunately, we tend to do this much less than most children. Be sure that you don't mislead yourself.

For goals to play a vital role in your motivation for exercise, they must be achievable. If and when they are accomplished, and if proper reinforcement is then forthcoming, skill learning and execution, and ultimately, level of fitness will be enhanced. But if your stated goal is nothing more than an expression of bravado or wishful thinking, then its chances of being realized are very slim. Thus, your ambition to continue with the exercise program will be weakened.

When you set exercise goals, be certain of their achievability. It's better to slightly undershoot a goal in the beginning than to set it too high. Once again I feel obliged to offer the reminder that we are no longer 20 or 25 years of age. Therefore, don't extract from your substantial memory bank of yesteryear's physical feats—efforts and achievements that are no longer within your repertoire. Think about what you can accomplish now! Think realistically—and set your exercise goals accordingly.

Having said this, let me offer one more piece of advice about goal setting: Once you're on the way, when you've actually begun your program, set your exercise goals as high as realism permits. The higher the better. Once you've launched your program, you can ratchet up the degree of difficulty as long as realism remains your guide.

In the long run, goals that challenge you result in better performance, better training, and better outcomes. At the outset, a conservative approach is best. Later on, as your aerobic capacity, muscular strength and endurance, agility, and flexibility attain higher levels, and as your psychological framework is secure, you can reset your exercise goals and make them more demanding.

Which brings us to yet another important point: As you move forward with your exercise program, keep assessing your progress; keep seeking feedback from your body. Continually test the levels of your fitness elements and as they improve, modify your goals. How does your body feel? Are your legs less heavy after your walk in comparison to how they felt last month? When you kayak or row, do you feel less discomfort in arm and shoulder muscles?

Good goal setting involves changeability. Don't fear changing your fitness goals. In fact, systematic reestablishment of expected exercise outcomes should be part of your overall strategy. Don't lose sight of the fact that the goals you set are yours and yours alone. Take possession of them and accept them. Difficulty along these lines may suggest errors in goal setting. If you have trouble taking ownership, if you can't proclaim complete possession of the goals you've set, reconsider their appropriateness. Maybe you are demanding too much or too little of yourself. *In addition to being realistic, be honest. Don't hesitate to admit that your originally established goals are faulty.* When necessary, modify them.

Don't lend your personal goals to anyone, and by all means, don't borrow goals from someone else. Appropriate goals are custom made for you; they are yours alone.

☞ WHAT YOU'VE LEARNED IN THIS CHAPTER

In this chapter the spotlight was upon goal setting. Goals are statements of fitness-training outcomes that you plan to achieve. These statements should be recorded and posted in a prominent location. From time to time they should be inspected and reconsidered. And above all, they should be realistic and attainable. They should incorporate challenge, but at the outset of your fitness program they may be less demanding than they are likely to be later on when your motivational foundation is well established.

Goals are highly personal in that they accommodate your own fitness levels and aspire to further develop fitness components. They belong to you and are not transferable to friends, colleagues, and even others who may be members of your exercise group or class.

Another aspect of proper goal setting is your readiness to embark upon a fitness training program. Think about your degree of preparedness to get started. If you are not ready, then even the best laid plans or the most carefully thought-out goals will not yield desired consequences. In this chapter I recommend a series of questions that will help you assess your readiness.

Goals should be realistic and systematically evaluated in order to be sure that they still reflect sensible fitness targets. Seek information from your body—your legs, arms, lungs, ligaments, and tendons. Ask them, "How're you doing?" They will provide answers. Listen to their responses and use them as a basis for altering your goals.

Establish short- as well as long-term goals. Each and every workout should be guided by goals. And goals should be established for weeks, months, and even years in advance. Make your exercise goals as specific as possible. In this chapter I provide examples of well-stated and poorly stated goals.

When done properly, goals setting will strengthen your motivation for sticking with your exercise program.

FOOD FOR THOUGHT
1 Are you ready to begin an exercise program? Is now a good time?
2 What kind of program can you presently embark upon in terms of available equipment, facilities, and time? Consider these issues carefully. If you are not quite ready, so be it. Perhaps in a little while your answers to these questions will reflect a stronger preparedness to begin.
3 Take a look at other exercisers. Chat with them, and notice the strength of their commitment and level of motivation. Examine the doses and intensities of their activities, and judge whether they have established realistic and attainable goals.
4 Determine if a correlation or connection exists between the fitness levels of exercisers you know and their use of goal setting. Are the goal setters in better shape than those who exercise without established targets?

Chapter 9

CHOOSING THE RIGHT EXERCISES FOR YOU

I'm 65 years old and overweight. My kids, grandkids, doctor, and husband all encourage me to take some exercise, but I don't know what to do. I read all about the importance of being physically active, but running marathons is not for me. Basketball is not for me, nor is lifting heavy weights. And I'm embarrassed to put on a pair of skimpy gym shorts and go to a health club. What do I do? Where and how do I begin?

Despite your serious intentions and sky-high level of enthusiasm, if you're about to tackle a program of exercise, particularly after years of inactivity, you require guidance. Your selection of activities and intensity of exercise should be influenced by principles and guidelines that take into consideration your readiness to begin. You are entering your golden years—a truly wonderful time of life. If you select activities that are inappropriate, not only will the desired results enumerated throughout this book be elusive, but you may also set the stage for injury.

In the preceding chapters I've talked time and time again about *sensible exercise*, and this chapter is all about helping you develop and apply this principle. Even when done with regularity and zeal, if the activities are wrong for you, they are

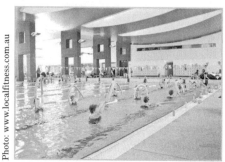

Photo: www.localfitness.com.au

We are all different people. Our body types are different, our movements are different, our health is different—we even have preferences to different sport. It's important to choose the right exercise that works for *you*.

without merit and potentially harmful. I can't comment upon every possible kind of physical activity, but I can provide recommendations designed to help you make suitable exercise choices.

But first,—congratulations are in order. If you've reached this point in the book, you probably have more than a passing interest in exercise. You may very well be in the third stage of the Transtheoretical Model described in Chapter 7. You may be ready to establish and enter an exercise program that's right for you, that's sensible and safe.

Here are four essential general principles to abide by when planning your personal exercise program.

Principle 1: *Develop a clear understanding of your individual and particular needs.*

All of us share some common exercise goals, but you undoubtedly have a set that is predicated upon your exclusive activity requirements. Consider the following categories of typical personal needs and prioritize them; by all means, add any that you believe are important:

- weight regulation
- muscular endurance
- muscular strength
- balance enhancement
- agility and flexibility enhancement
- cardio respiratory efficiency

What's number one on your list? And what evidence justifies this ranking? What is it that enables you to conclude that one or two of the above categories require particular attention? How do you know that you are overweight or low in muscular strength?

Have legitimate assessment procedures been conducted by qualified professionals in order to determine the amount of body fat you store or the appropriateness of your total body weight in proportion to your skeletal frame and height? If you've given cardiorespiratory efficiency a high priority, what's the basis for your judgment? Has your physician determined that you are deficient in this area, or is your evaluation based exclusively upon your intuition? Have you been checked out for cardiovascular disease that may be present despite the superficial appearance of your perceived sound health?

Don't be surprised if your perception of a paramount need or strength doesn't jibe with your physician's opinion. Are you sure that your prioritization is accurate? On a scale of 1–10, what number represents your level of certainty? If the number is below 7, chances are that you need expert advice. Where can you get such help? This book should serve as a good source of relevant information. But you have to be a part of the decision making. So the first step is to consider your recreational interests and how they relate to your various fitness components (strengths and weaknesses).

If you see yourself as being a bit shy on the agility, and sailing is your cup of tea, then a perceived low ranking in this category may not be much of a problem. However, if folk dancing is something you wish to pursue as exercise, then you should consider shoring up the agility component of your fitness. Continuing in this vein, gardening requires that your muscular endurance be reasonably high because you would be using arm movements repetitively. Your back muscles would also be heavily involved. On the other hand, if it's swimming that captures your fancy, then you'll require substantial cardio respiratory endurance. And a good deal of heavy resistance training for the upper body would probably not be necessary if you select golf as your primary recreational/fitness activity, although some weight lifting with light weights might be of benefit in order to strengthen certain muscle groups essential to a correct swing. Above all, remember: regardless of your recreational preference, a wholesome exercise program includes some effort in each of the fitness categories. You should definitely incorporate some degree of strength, endurance, agility, flexibility, etc., training in your regimen.

Perhaps your primary motivation for entering an exercise program is not focused narrowly upon any recreational interest. Sport may not be something that interests you. The very thought of competition turns you off. This is fine. It is entirely appropriate for your motivation to revolve around maintenance of optimal health and well being.

This being the case, examine your typical everyday physical challenges and assignments, such as walking to the bus stop, vacuuming the carpet, taking the trash cans to the top of the driveway, raking leaves in the yard, climbing stairs, cutting grass, shoveling snow, or lifting a young niece, nephew, or grandchild. These would be activities in which you are involved frequently or even on a regular basis.

Now pose and answer this question: Are you able to satisfy the physical requirements of each of these activities without undue difficulty? As you think about these things, perhaps one fitness dimension is revealed to be a trifle below par and in need of adjustment. This insight then becomes part of the decision-making strategy as you plan your exercise program. The idea is to ask the right questions and provide honest answers (see Chapter 8). Another such important question is: To what extent am I prepared to begin a program? What exactly is my state of readiness? Am I primed and raring to go, or am I still merely contemplating starting an exercise regimen? Am I presently doing some physical activity, or am I completely sedentary? Am I ready for a change? Table 9.2 will assist you in getting a grip on these issues.

Principle 2: *If your program is based on recreational interests, then be sure to incorporate movements that closely resemble actions inherent in the activities for which you are preparing.*

Make sure that the agility or strength training movements in your exercise regimen parallel as much as possible the authentic movements in your anticipated recreational activity. If you are preparing for snow skiing, simulate the large-muscle action basically required in this activity. Tennis involves considerable activation of wrist, shoulder, back, and leg muscles. Be sure to somehow include these muscle groups when constructing your exercise regimen.

If you are interested in an elevated overall level of fitness, then integrate all fitness components when establishing your program. Attend to each of the enumerated categories (agility, flexibility, muscular strength, etc.) and be sure to incorporate at least a few movements that ensure coverage of all bases. Have a look at Table 9.1 to get information about which muscles are involved in various kinds of physical activities as well as the extent of aerobic, agility, and flexibility emphases.

Principle 3: *Be realistic in configuring your program.*
Don't commit to something that you will be unlikely to sustain for an appreciable length of time. If your program is unrealistically ambitious you run the risk of dropping out despite your good intentions. Be authentic and reasonable in listing your aspirations (see Chapter 8). Don't permit your enthusiasm to override rational and safe thinking and planning. Although you may move well and are capable of notable physical accomplishments, you are no longer 16. Don't make decisions about exercise that would befit a teenager.

Three Ss should serve as reminders: Be *smart, sincere,* and *safe.* And three Rs should also be helpful: Be *realistic, responsible,* and *respectful* of your body's abilities.

Lastly, be sure to assess your progress periodically to be assured that the work prescriptions you've undertaken are appropriate. Monitor your fatigue during exercise, as well as the amount of effort you've expended. Ask yourself two straightforward questions and answer them honestly:

1. How am I doing?

2. Am I making progress in comparison to last month and last week?

Table. 9. 1. Muscles Involved in Various Physical Activities

Activity	Primary muscle groups involved	Aerobic emphasis	Strength and muscular endurance emphases	Flexibility and agility emphases
Archery	Arms, chest, back (upper), hands	No	Yes	Flexibility—yes, agility—no
Ballroom dancing	Upper and lower body, feet	Yes—moderate to high	Yes—moderate	Yes—very high
Bowling	Dominant arm and hand, legs, thighs	No	Yes—moderate	Yes—moderate
Canoeing	Upper body, arms, hands, abdominal	Yes—high	Yes—high	Flexibility—moderate, agility—no
Folk dancing	Upper and lower body, feet	Yes—high	Yes—both—moderate	Yes—both—high
Golf	All muscles of back and arms	No	Yes—moderate	Yes—low to moderate
Horseshoe pitching	Upper body—dominant side	No	Yes—moderate	No
Jogging	Legs, feet, abdominal	Yes—high	Yes—moderate to high	No
Rowing	Upper body, arms, hands, legs, abdominal	Yes—high	Yes—high	No
Skating	Legs, abdominal, feet, lower body, back	Yes—high	Yes—high	Yes—low to moderate
Skiing	Shoulders, back, lower body, hands, abdominal	Yes—high	Yes—high	Yes—moderate to high
Square dancing	Lower body, feet	Yes—low to moderate	Yes—moderate	Yes—moderate
Tennis	Upper body of dominant side, dominant hand forearm, arm	Yes—low to moderate	Yes—moderate	Yes—high

Table. 9. 1. (Continued).				
Activity	Primary muscle groups involved	Aerobic emphasis	Strength and muscular endurance emphases	Flexibility and agility emphases
Rock climbing	All large skeletal muscles, shoulders, all limbs, both hands and feet, neck	Yes—high	Yes—high	Yes—moderate to high
Volleyball	Upper body, legs, hands, feet	Yes—low to moderate	Yes—low	Yes—moderate
Walking/ hiking	Upper and lower body, feet	Yes—moderate to high	Yes—low	No

Don't hesitate to admit that the assignments you've undertaken are inappropriate. Be willing and prepared to make necessary adjustments. Reconfigure your FIT components.

Principle 4: *Three types of exercise should definitely be incorporated into your regular exercise routines but with varying emphases, depending upon your goals, needs, and fitness objectives. These three types are* stretching, resistance, *and* aerobic exercise.

STRETCHING

Function of your large skeletal muscles is benefited when you stretch both prior to (warm up) and after (cool down) exercising. Stretching prepares muscles for strenuous physical activity by loosening them. Don't be misled by advice to the contrary. Some published research suggests that elite sprinters who stretch before competing experience the same frequency of injury as in those who do not stretch. My assumption is that you are not in this category. No offense intended, but the likelihood of you being an elite competitive sprinter at the collegiate or international level is small. Especially at your age.

Table 9.2. Physical Activity History

If you do not currently participate in physical activity, answer these questions:

1. How long has it been since you did *regular* physical activity or exercise?

    a. less than 6 months
    b. more than 6 months but less than 1 year
    c. more than 1 but less than 2 years
    d. more than 2 but less than 5 years
    e. more than 5 but less than 10 years
    f. more than 10 years
    g. I have never been regularly physically active

If you are currently physically active answer the following questions:

1. How many days are you physically active?
2. Approximately how many minutes are you physically active each time?
3. How long have you been physically active at this level?
4. What activities do you do?

Answer the following questions whether or not you are currently physically active.

1. As an adult, were there ever times when you were physically active regularly for at least three months and then stopped being physically active for at least three months?
2. If yes, how many times?
3. Regarding the most recent time, why did you stop your activity? (Please check as many as apply.)

    Lack of time because of:

work or school	lack of physical activity partner
household duties	lack of interest in physical activity
children	health problems
social activities	injury
spouse	season or weather change
lack of money	personal stress
lack of facilities	other

From B. H. Marcus and L. H. Forsyth, 2009, *Motivating people to be physically active*, 2nd ed. (Champaign, IL: Human Kinetics), 176.

Try to isolate the specific muscles and muscle groups that you believe will be activated during your resistance and aerobic routines. *Don't bounce while stretching* because bouncing creates a counteraction that actually results in muscle tightening. Stretch slowly (*statically*) to a point of mild discomfort, but not pain. Hold the stretch for about 20 seconds and repeat three times for each muscle group. If time permits, stretch at the beginning of your program or before you start your activity, as well as at the end.

You'll probably find it easier to stretch at the end of your routine or activity because at this point your muscle temperature is higher, which means that your muscles are looser. As your stretched skeletal muscles loosen, your tolerance for any discomfort associated with the stretch should increase. You'll thus be able to hold the stretch a bit longer.

Some experts recommend that *dynamic stretching* (not stretching of the very slow and sustained variety, but for example, stretching that involves effortful movement of limbs such as in kicking) be done prior to exercise and *static stretching* be the choice at the conclusion of the exercise.

Some of the advice I've just offered is at the moment somewhat controversial. Experts are not in complete accord about the best times to stretch dynamically or statically. If in doubt, go with the static stretch before as well as after exercise.

The gurus disagree somewhat about the time requirement for the stretch. Some advocate a particular number of seconds (I've indicated above that about 20 seconds is sufficient). Others insist that time itself is not of essence. They speak of the need to reach the *point of zero tension* before stopping. This point varies from muscle group to muscle group as well as individual to individual. I refer you once again to a book I recommended in Chapter 5 that provides detailed descriptions of this and other controversies involving stretching: *The Stark Reality of Stretching,* by Dr. Steven Stark.

PILATES AND YOGA

Two currently popular exercise protocols that incorporate a good deal of stretching are *Pilates* and *yoga*. The former is an exercise format that involves very controlled movements with an emphasis on strengthening of the *core muscles* (those that connect to the spinal cord, rib cage, and pelvis). In addition, it highlights body awareness, which is an important ingredient of injury prevention (see Chapter 5). If you maintain an awareness of where your body and its parts are located in space, your control of the body is more precise and the probability of injury is thus reduced.

Yoga is a form of exercise that is essentially concerned with improving strength and flexibility. It utilizes postures performed slowly and quickly. In my view both yoga and Pilates should be supplemented with some sort of aerobic exercise in order to assure a comprehensive approach to fitness. Advocates and practitioners of yoga speak highly of its capacities to improve balance and reduce stress.

Stretch it!

RESISTANCE MOVEMENTS

When your skeletal muscles contract against loads that increase progressively over weeks and months, they respond by increasing in size and strength. Some exceptions to this generalization exist, but more often than not, this is the case. And such is the basis for what is commonly known as *weight lifting* or *weight training*.

Maintaining or improving your muscular strength should be an important objective of your fitness training, because most muscles lose some of their abilities to overcome resistance (lifting, pushing, etc.) during adult aging. I'm aware that I've made the following observation before, but it merits repetition: You are no longer of an age when vigorous resistance training would yield the kind of results that it would have some 40 years ago, so expect impressive but not overwhelming results. You no longer have the hormones necessary for increasing the girth of skeletal musculature to the same degree as when you were in your teens or early 20s. Therefore, your goals should change commensurately.

Your primary goal now is to maintain as much of your development as feasible or to improve it to whatever extent possible (a good example of exercise sensibility). *Muscular atrophy* is what you're up against, and your aim is to slow down this regrettable but unavoidable process. Take solace in knowing that studies using men in their 80s and 90s have shown that very real improvement in strength can occur as a result of weight training, but, of course, not to the same extent as in subjects who are in their teens and early to mid-20s. You can benefit significantly now from resistance training even if you've never done it before.

Although strength and endurance are not the same, use of the same training objectives for them both makes sense. *Endurance* refers to the ability of the muscle or muscle group to sustain a contraction over a relatively long period of time or to repeat the contraction over and over again. When you do sit-ups or push-ups you are testing the *endurance* of muscles in your chest and arms. When you lift a heavy weight once, you are demonstrating *muscular strength.* For endurance training use relatively light weights and repeat the movement a minimum of six times. Use heavier loads for strength training.

Barbells and machines found in gymnasia are designed to provide safe and convenient strength and endurance exercise, but you can also utilize materials you have at home. An unopened can of soup or a one-gallon jug of water provides adequate resistance for your arm or shoulder muscles, at least in the beginning of your program. A tennis ball squeezed repetitively is an effective apparatus for hand and forearm endurance development (tennis grip).

If you are getting your strength and endurance exercise through sport activities, analyze the basic movements involved to determine if you are incorporating endurance and strength aspects of your fitness goals. Introduce modifications when necessary. For example, walking involves many repetitions of leg extension and hip and ankle flexion while challenging your body to move its own weight in space. But it's shy on activation of arm and upper body muscles. So carry something while you walk. A stone that fits comfortably in your grip or a tote bag that you can shift from one hand to the other every few minutes will do nicely. Think creatively, experiment, and figure out how to provide resistance.

List all large skeletal muscles in the limbs, upper body, and lower body (don't be concerned with assigning correct anatomical names), and without employing any resistance beyond the weight of the body part, determine what movements seem to activate them. Then determine how much weight (for example, a one-gallon water jug or smaller can of soup) you can handle as you try to move the body part or limb through space. In this manner devise a series of resistance exercises for all large muscle groups. Use your body weight itself as resistance. Lie on your back with feet together and raise both heels simultaneously off the floor to activate abdominal muscles. (This is only an example of how to employ the weight of your own body, but be careful about placing too much strain on you abdominal wall too soon.)

Some muscles will be more difficult to isolate than others, and some groups will require more creative use of household materials. The critical thing is to know how much you can safely handle. One of the advantages of using health club or gym facilities is that the machines and weighted implements are designed to let you move resistances safely. A second advantage is that you are able to easily quantify the amount of resistance used by simply reading the amount of weight indicated on the plate or whatever else the device employs.

Lift it!

AEROBIC EXERCISE

When you inspire environmental air during exercise, the activity is called *aerobic*. Walking, jogging, skiing, and swimming above the water's surface with proper technique are examples. When your breath is held, as in underwater swimming, and you rely on oxygen already stored in your body to provide fuel and energy needed for muscular exertion, your efforts are said to be *anaerobic* (without air). If you lift a large weight by first taking a substantial gulp of air and then close our mouth, you are performing anaerobically.

Your exercise program should definitely incorporate some aerobic activities. Be sure to include walking (treadmill walking and mall walking are fine), jogging, swimming, or bicycle riding for about 20–30 minutes, three times a week. Rowing, either in a real, on-the-water setting or with a gymnasium rowing machine, is an excellent aerobic exercise. By all means, pursue bowling, horseshoe pitching, heavy resistance training, archery, golf, bocce, or whatever constitutes your heart's desire. But be sure to incorporate some sort of aerobic exercise in your program. Boomers should place a decided accent upon two components of fitness training in particular: flexibility and aerobic exercise.

Now that I've established some general exercise principles let's move on to details that are a bit more specific. The following guidelines should be helpful in selecting your most appropriate physical activities.

Guidelines for Selecting the Right Exercises: Things to Bear in Mind When Constructing Your Program

IN THE GYM OR HEALTH CLUB

1. With your targeted body areas in mind try to cover as many muscle groups as possible. Use a checklist so that no important group is omitted from your exercise plan. Identify lower and upper body muscle groups. Again, don't be concerned about applying their correct names. For instance, use terms such as *shoulder*, *front* or *back of arm*, *calf*, *front of thigh*, or *abdominal area* (*abdominal area* is a better term than *stomach* because the latter is an internal organ, which is not what you're targeting), *neck*, *upper back*, *lower back*. Use available resources such as a high school biology book or anatomy chart in your physician's waiting room, or plug *muscle* into your favorite internet search engine to determine correct movements for each. Personal trainers at gyms can help. Books and references provided in the reference section of this book can advise as to exactly how to perform each of many appropriate exercises.

2. *Exercise machines* can be costly but have advantages over free weights or use of your body itself as the source of resistance. Machines provide a margin of safety in that you are compelled to move your limbs and torso in highly prescribed directions. In a manner of speaking, your movements are patterned or restricted. The machine permits you only to extend the arm or flex the knee within a very narrow range of motion. Therefore, the potential for self-abuse and injury is minimized. And you can't drop a heavy weight or soup can on your foot accidentally.

There's also the matter of convenience. If you wish to increase or decrease the amount of resistance against which your muscles will contract, you have but to relocate a pin that will determine the amount of plates on the machine to be activated. You can purchase all-purpose exercise machines for home use. By all-purpose, I mean devices that will enable you to bring a large number of muscle groups into play by changing your grip and position (standing, sitting, etc.) or manipulating some part of the machine itself. Resistance training need not incorporate dumbbells or fancy weight machinery. A variety of very helpful devices can be used at home or when you travel. Large rubber bands with handles, springs with handles, or even your own body weight can become objects of resistance.

Gymnasiums, be they in health clubs, YMCAs, or community recreational facilities open to the public, usually contain arrays of exercise machines. Try them out and get the feel of them before signing up for membership. Determine how many machines there are of each kind because during peak hours they tend to be heavily used and you may end up waiting for a turn. Most modern gymnasiums are also equipped with treadmills, stationary bicycles, rowing machines, mechanisms that simulate stair climbing, and gliders (also known as elliptical machines) that permit you to slide your feet as if you were cross-country skiing. This reduces, or practically eliminates, the skeletal shock inherent in running.

3. Plan on doing three sets of each of your selected exercises. After completing one set of 6–12 repetitions at a particular

station, move on to an adjacent machine or to your next exercise but return to it later for your second and third sets. You should do three sets. A single set consists of the aforementioned 6–12 repetitions or *reps*. In the interim, move on to other machines. If you move quickly from one machine to another or actually jog, you can incorporate an adequate measure of aerobic training in your regimen.

Circuit training is a method that relies on the rapid execution (in good form, of course) of each exercise, followed by a hustle to the next machine or exercise station. Circuit training need not be used exclusively with machines but can also be done with each station representing some form of calisthenics, such as sit-ups, push-ups, pull-ups, lunges, etc., where your body weight is the source of resistance. Circuit training gives priority to rapid execution of the three sets (proper form must not be sacrificed). Progress is measured not only in terms of how much resistance you overcome at each station (how much weight you can handle on the machine or where you set the pin), but how much time is necessary to complete all three sets or circuits.

After a few weeks of training, the total amount of time should decrease, thereby indicating an improvement in muscular strength, muscular endurance, and cardiorespiratory fitness, depending on the type of movements or exercises you've incorporated at each station. You'll need a watch or better yet, a stopwatch to monitor your achievement. A helpful way to assess the effectiveness of your circuit training efforts would be to time yourself for a brief walk or jog prior to embarking upon the program and then, three weeks after training, do the same. The amount of time needed to complete the walk or jog should decrease.

I've used circuit training as a personal form of exercise as well as in classes I've taught over the years. I've found it to be an excellent system for fostering all dimensions of fitness, including aerobic capacity. It can be done even in the most limited living space by incorporating movements that don't require elaborate apparatus. It's also a good option when traveling. Do a circuit in your hotel room by incorporating movements that depend only on the space and equipment (chairs, carpet) in the environment. If done at home, use chairs for dips or any other piece of furniture that lends itself to exercise by enabling you to move your body against gravity. Just move quickly and execute all components of the program absolutely correctly.

On the Track, Treadmill, or Road

Walking, jogging, or running are common ways to satisfy the aerobic requirement of your exercise program, although as I've mentioned previously, other forms, such as cycling, swimming, rowing, skiing, and skating are excellent alternatives. But running, jogging, and walking require no fancy or expensive equipment, and therefore, you may find them to be good choices. Moreover, locations for jogging or walking are much more readily available than ice rinks, ski slopes, lakes, rivers, or even swimming pools.

If you are a cycling enthusiast, you are obliged to have your bike handy wherever you may be. You have to take it with you when traveling or arrange to borrow or rent one. But a suitable location for your walk or jog is usually available in almost any venue. If staying in a hotel, ask the bellhop to advise as to where walking or jogging is safe and the vistas or scenery attractive. Mind you, I'm by no means disparaging any of the above activities, for they are all excellent forms of aerobic conditioning. I'm merely suggesting that walking, jogging, or running don't require the facilities necessary for the other aerobic activities. I also realize that special concerns such as knee or foot problems may be good reasons for excluding walking, running, or jogging. This brings us back to cycling.

Riding is easier on the knees than jogging or fast walking and new kinds of bicycles have recently come on the market that have made riding bikes less of a challenge to stability. Three-wheelers are readily available for those with balance problems. Helmets are a must for cyclists because they are almost 90% effective in preventing brain injuries. And above all, when riding on the road, ride with traffic, not against it.

Ride it!

If You're Going to Walk, Hike, Jog, or Run:

1. Wear appropriate footwear. Don't skimp on good walking or jogging shoes. Spend a little more and purchase well-cushioned and supportive footwear. Find another way to save money. Buy good shoes for exercising, particularly for jogging, running, or walking. If your feet tend to pronate (turn in or come down on the inner margin of the foot) purchase shoes with a straight last (minimum curve of the sole). If you are inclined to supinate (hit the ground with the outermost or outside edge of the foot), a curved last should be your choice.

2. Be wary of the sun. Wear a hat with a brim that offers adequate protection. Use sun block and use it liberally. Wear sunglasses after 10 a.m.

3. Hydrate (drink water) before embarking upon your run or jog. Take some water with you and don't hesitate to imbibe as you exercise. This caution also applies to swimming and cycling. Swimmers usually don't realize that they perspire and lose water while exercising. But it's true, so hydrate before swimming. Clip a water bottle onto your bike and drink at will. The days are long gone when drinking water during, before, or after exercise was considered sissy stuff.

4. Be careful about terrain and surfaces upon which you'll exercise. Rubberized track surfaces that many high school and local college tracks have installed are excellent for shock absorption. If park or forest trails appeal to you, be wary of stones and fallen limbs that may be strewn in the pathway. Think about such obstacles when deciding upon a location for your activity. Consider the safety of your intended walking, running, or jogging route. Some neighborhoods and parks may be less safe than others.

5. Be conservative when constructing your program. Don't start out with a bang lest you be injured, discomforted, or discouraged. Don't be overly ambitious. If you are uncertain about your capacity, underestimate how far you should walk or jog. You can always increase the distance after a while. If

you have difficulty in talking while jogging or walking, you are moving too fast.

6. Exercise aerobically on a regular basis. Three times a week will suffice in the beginning. After gaining confidence in your body's ability to handle related demands, you can add a day or two.

7. Be cautious about increasing the distance you cover in your walk, jog, or run. A good rule of thumb is, *no more than 10% of an increase in distance every two weeks*. If you've been jogging about a mile, after about two weeks try moving up to about a mile and one tenth. See how it goes.

8. Back off if you feel nagging fatigue or you sense that your aerobic exercise is becoming a burden. Give yourself permission to rest for a day. It's okay. Over a period of a few weeks, after cultivating a decent level of aerobic capacity, you're entitled to a day off. You won't lose any gained aerobic advantage if you return to your regimen after a brief layoff. In fact a day or two of rest will provide more benefit than harm; being obstinate and making yourself vulnerable to injury can be an unnecessary consequence (see Chapter 5).

   Avoid being a martinet. Leave martyrdom for the professional athletes. Sometimes inclement weather can provide an opportunity for rest. Don't hesitate to take occasional advantage of such circumstances. Many joggers and walkers like to listen to music while exercising. If you plug in earphones while jogging, be mindful of hazards like traffic and other persons in the environment. When listening to music or talk radio while engaged in physical activity, you are multitasking and may not be reacting to or coping with important environmental stimuli.

9. Consider a currently popular approach to pursuing aerobic fitness known as *cross training*. This involves alternating two or three different kinds of aerobic activity during the course of a week. For instance, on Monday you would jog; on Tuesday you would walk. On Wednesday you'd walk again, and on Thursday you might swim, ride the stationary

bike, or cycle outside. By changing the activities you rest primary muscle groups yet tax your cardiorespiratory mechanisms. Another advantage of cross training is that, over the long haul, you can avoid boredom or *staleness*.

WHAT'S THE DIFFERENCE BETWEEN JOGGING AND RUNNING?

Although elite race walkers can move faster than you and I can jog or perhaps even run, as a rule, walking and jogging involve slower action than running. I consider anything faster than an eight minute per mile pace to be running. Moving slower is jogging or walking. A speed between 15 to 20 minutes per mile is more than adequate for fitness walking. Slower than a 20-minute pace is *strolling*, by all means a legitimate recreational activity and one that will provide some cardiorespiratory and leg muscle pay-off. If you move at precisely a 20-minute pace, in an hour you'll cover three miles, a very reasonable and safe objective for the beginner. Don't be in a rush.

Believe it or not, the aerobic benefit derived from walking and jogging doesn't differ much from that provided by running. I've always believed that in terms of caloric cost, greater caloric expenditure could be demonstrated in the scientific laboratory for running rather than walking, but in the real world in which you and I operate, the difference is not very meaningful. You burn almost as many calories during a jog as during a run. And a brisk walk at a pace of 14 or 15 minutes a mile pace comes in a close third. This was my belief for many years; however, after coming across a piece in the December 2009 issue of the University of California, Berkley *Wellness Letter* I'm inclined to modify my opinion. I believe a direct quote from this reference would be informative and helpful here:

> Do you burn more calories if you run or if you briskly walk it? Many people claim you'd use the same number of calories, because you're transporting the same amount of weight over the same distance. It's a law of physics, they say, and if you run, you just burn the calories faster.

This belief is widespread, according to our research on
the internet. But it is not true. It's not just that it takes
more energy to move your body at higher speed, but running also requires more strenuous arm, leg, and upper-
body movement, and it raises your heart rate more, all of
which burn extra calories. And to achieve the longer stride
of running, you have to repeatedly lift your body weight
off the ground so that both feet are in the air at the same
time. When you walk, at least one foot is always on the
ground. Race-walking, with its hip-swiveling, arm-
pumping motion, also burns more calories per mile than
regular walking.

A standard reference guide to energy expenditures
shows that for a 132-pound person, walking three miles
per hour burns, on average, 70 calories per mile (in 20 minutes), but running 6 miles per hour burns 100 calories per
mile (in 10 minutes). And in a 2004 study, researchers from
Syracuse University measured energy expenditures in 24
people and found that running a mile on a track or treadmill takes 30% more calories than walking it at half speed.

Brisk walking is still a great way to burn calories, and
many people prefer it to running, in part because it is easier on the body. But if you want to burn as many calories
as you would running, you have to walk farther. (p. 6)

Of course, if you desire to prepare for road racing or competitive walking, you'd be obliged to train through fast walking or
running. This is necessary mostly to condition skeletal muscles,
ligaments, and tendons involved in relatively faster movements
and to stress on your cardiovascular system a little more. By
the way, don't discount competitive walking or running.

Road races can be a lot of fun if your mind-set is appropriate. The fact that they usually acknowledge age categories enables Boomers and even considerably older participants to establish very realistic and safe competitive goals. When you
enter one of the popular 5K or 10K Saturday morning road
races that I'm sure your community or neighboring community occasionally sponsors as a fundraiser for a worthy cause,

you strive to excel over runners of your same sex and age. The medal goes to the first place male and female finisher in the 60–64 age bracket or 65–69 age group.

These events can provide a nice reward for your weeks or months of adherence to your aerobic training program. You're a winner if you just finish. So why not let finishing be your personal goal (see Chapter 8). Or determine that you want to complete the 5K event (3.1 miles) in something sensible, like 40–45 minutes. And if you bring a friend, partner, spouse, and/or grandkids to cheer you on as you cross the finish line, you not only benefit from the inspiration and motivation they engender but also enable the morning to be a pleasant experience for your own little group of cheerleaders. The same opportunities are often available for swimmers, cyclists, skiers, and tennis players.

Move it!

IN THE WATER

In my experience, Boomers who undertake swimming as their mode of regular exercise usually have some sort of background in the activity. By no means is this the case with all who chose swimming, and it's certainly not the case with those who prefer other aquatic activities such as water skiing or sailing. But these are my observations. Boomers who swim competitively often swam as high school or college athletes and are now returning to the water. An absolutely great idea!

Having said this, let me provide assurance that I know more than a few regular swimmers over the age of 60 who never swam competitively, and still don't. They swim for aerobic benefit or because the water's buoyancy enables them to avoid the skeletal jarring inherent in jogging, running, and many of the racket and ball sports. The pool (or lake, river, and ocean, when feasible) frees them from problems associated with the automobile traffic and hazards of the road. For them, the routine of lap after lap in the same lane and its potential tedium is more than adequately counterbalanced by the much valued privacy and substantial profit to the cardiorespiratory system. Once again, do your own thing. Acknowledge your personal needs, likes, dislikes, and interests.

In terms of providing aerobic benefit, canoeing, kayaking, and similar water activities easily fit the bill. In fact, they do more than merely accomplish this. In addition, they present excellent opportunities for developing muscular strength and endurance. The upper body skeletal musculature, in particular, is soundly activated and challenged during these activities.

But these activities are quite expensive in comparison to running, jogging, walking, and probably swimming. Boats have to be either purchased or rented. Transportation to and from the river or lake is also a consideration. And prevailing weather conditions influence the frequency for participation. You can walk, jog, or run indoors (indoor tracks or the shopping mall for walking, for instance). Indoor participation is not feasible for canoeing and kayaking and similar activities.

Another consideration in comparing these boating activities to walking, jogging, or running is the level of skill required to participate. If you are organically and structurally sound, you are hard-wired for walking and jogging. If you are in some way mobility challenged, you can still walk with support (cane, walker, crutches). If you are a neophyte canoeist or kayaker, you'll need instruction. Don't go on the water alone the first few times.

Sailing is another matter altogether. One doesn't simply declare intent to sail recreationally or for reasons of fitness. This is not to say it's out of the question as a fitness activity, because some persons may indeed have the necessary financial resources, time, and skill at their disposal. Sailing provides many different kinds of fitness and recreational opportunities because different kinds of vessels demand different sets of skills and experiences. Some have a formidable aerobic component, some do not, but instead emphasize cognitive and navigational skills.

Swim it!

Other Exercise Options

I've enumerated but a few common exercise activities in this chapter. Obviously many more exist, but they don't necessarily involve substantial aerobic challenge. Activities such as bowling, golf, croquet, curling (popular among the Canadians), gardening, archery, and shooting are fine activities and will satisfy many of your physical needs. Bocce has become very popular in the last few years and is attracting more and more older participants. These activities comprise wonderful recreational, diversionary, and fitness opportunities, but their emphases are decidedly not aerobic.

Unfortunately, in a book such as this it is unreasonable to anticipate complete coverage of all conceivable recreational/ sport aerobic activities. Rock climbing, for instance, is a demanding aerobic activity that offers ardent participants high level fitness training opportunities from almost all perspectives. However, it's an example of one exercise/recreational experience that I'll not be able to talk about because the book's number of pages and word count are realistic concerns that I'm obliged to deal with.

And I'm sure that there are many others you've heard of or have in mind depending upon your cultural heritage and geographic location. So don't conclude that if a particular activity is not listed here that it's out of the question. Just consider the guidelines and principles I've enumerated earlier and apply them to whatever activities you're contemplating. *Get started, and permit yourself to enjoy your exercise for any number of reasons.*

Organized Exercise Opportunities for Boomers

After having done your regular routine unfailingly for some time, you might wish to see to what extent your fitness and skill levels have improved or how you compare with others of your age and experience. Older people have a number of opportunities to gather, compete, socialize, or just exercise together and enjoy themselves enormously. See if any of the following appeal to you.

I'll provide information about available facilities and organizations that offer opportunities for men and women in their Boomer years to test their mettle through competition, meet others with similar exercise interests, or get ideas about alternate ways of pursuing their physical activity. You may not require such information. You may be content to pursue your established activity goals on your own. For some exercisers a chance to actually be alone is the day's highlight and the thought of sharing such delight with others is not at all attractive. But for those who feel such a need—here goes.

SILVER SNEAKERS

Silver Sneakers is a fitness program for older adults located in selected participating facilities (YMCAs, Gold's Gyms, retirement communities, etc.). Typical fare at almost any of the 3,000 locations nationwide are low-impact aerobics classes and exercises that incorporate light resistances (weights). The program has been adopted by health plans around the country for Medicare eligible folks and group retirees. Therefore, there's no cost to participants. Many health plans offer coverage. The average age of the men and women who are involved is about 70 years, and on a daily basis, approximately 60,000 exercisers participate. According to the Silver Sneakers literature, the first step to take is to determine which facilities in your area offer the program. Then you apply, fill out some paper work, and you're on your way to fun and fitness.

SENIOR GAMES

Every state in the union offers an annual "Games" wherein older persons are given the opportunity to perform in activities of their choice in competitive settings. Specific activities vary somewhat from state to state, but a common core of events is offered by most states. Participants must be no younger than 50 years of age and attend the Games at their own expense. Included in the schedule are social activities that enable involvement to be more than just an athletic assembly. The dates for your state's games will understandably be different than those posted by others. You can determine particulars by searching the internet if you are a computer user, or finding the appropriate telephone number in the Yellow Pages of you phone book.

NATIONAL SENIOR GAMES

For those who qualify, the annual National Senior Games, usually held in August, provides the chance to test their individual and team sport skills in comparison to others in their age group at a high level. Qualification entails being no younger than 50 years of age and having performed well at respective state senior games championships. The list of events is extensive: archery, badminton, basketball, bowling, cycling, golf, horseshoes, race walking, racquetball, road racing, shuffleboard, softball, swimming, table tennis, tennis, track and field, triathlon, volleyball, equestrian, fencing, lawn bowling, rowing, sailing, soccer, and water polo. Information can be obtained through the games' website—"Senior Games." Competitors must meet out-of-pocket travel and living expenses related to attending the games as well as registration fees.

YMCA

Founded in 1844, the Young Men's Christian Association now boasts some 14,000 locations in 122 countries throughout the world. Despite its religious grounding the Y welcomes members of all faiths, races, and ages. Activity programs vary from location to location, as each facility seeks to satisfy the needs and interests of those who live in the local community. Many of the locations offer the Silver Sneakers program described above, although members may partake of numerous other fitness and activity offerings. Many of the facilities have swimming pools and state-of-the-art exercise equipment. A membership fee is required. Many of the YMCA facilities have reciprocal arrangements with one another so that members who travel may avail themselves of exercise opportunities when on the road.

AMERICAN SENIOR FITNESS ASSOCIATION

This association exists for the purpose of training those individuals who wish to work with older exercisers. They offer various educational programs and certifications that many of the exercise programs available to older persons rely on for assurance that those they employ are appropriately prepared.

LOCAL SENIOR CENTERS

Many communities have within their boundaries a center dedicated to serving older persons. They typically present a full
range of physical activity options as well as crafts and different
kinds of interesting courses. Discussion groups, classes, and ex-
cursions are also often part of the fare.

☞ WHAT YOU'VE LEARNED IN THIS CHAPTER

This chapter provides guidelines and recommendations that
should enable you to tailor-make an exercise program that
caters to your individual needs and interests. You were encouraged to be realistic and safe and to properly assess any particular fitness dimensions that require special attention. In this
chapter you were urged to respect your body's abilities and not
hold unreasonable and unsafe expectations. In addition, the
importance of frequent assessment of progress, or lack thereof,
was emphasized so that you can reconfigure self-imposed assignments when necessary.

Three categories of exercise were described: *stretching, resistance*, and *aerobic exercise*. Your program should incorporate
activities from each area while acknowledging existing personal deficiencies. The activity program should undertake improvement in these weak spots where necessary. Advice was
given as to how to proceed with movements in each category.
For instance, with regard to stretching, you were encouraged
to avoid bouncing and to stop stretching until you feel pain.
With regard to resistance training (weight training), you learned
that no matter what your age, strength benefits await you if
you begin now.

The term *aerobic exercise* was defined and encouragement
provided as to the absolute need of including this type of exercise in every regimen. Boomers in particular should emphasize
aerobic as well as flexibility activities when constructing their
exercise programs.

Advantages to using exercise machines were discussed and
some recommendations made about how to incorporate these

devices into your program. Circuit training and cross training were described.

Hints were provided about maintaining safety while you partake of outdoor exercising. You learned about the importance of protecting your skin from the sun by using sunscreen and a hat. Specific advice about jogging and walking was also provided so that you might engage in these activities safely and profitably. Among the things you read about were pace and appropriate jogging or running speed. Exercise options on or in the water were reviewed and suggestions made.

Lastly, available organized opportunities for older exercisers and sport participants were described. These options may satisfy the interests of those who seek company and/or competition in the physical activities they've adopted as their exercise choices.

FOOD FOR THOUGHT

1	Have you noticed that areas of fitness that may be especially strong in your fitness profile may be in dire need of improvement in friends or acquaintances? What do you consider to be your fitness vulnerabilities?
2	In what ways(s) might your quality of life be enhanced if you were to significantly improve any of your fitness shortcomings?
3	After responding to the questions in Table 9.2, what do you conclude about your readiness to launch a physical activity program?
4	Do you appreciate how activities that you always considered to be recreational can be incorporated into exercise routines that satisfy basic fitness needs?

Epilogue: Final Food for Thought

My sincere hope is that you have profited in many ways from this book. First, your general knowledge about physical activity and its multitude of benefits to older persons should have been increased. You should now be conversant with many scientific terms that enable an understanding of why exercise is so important in your life. You have hopefully gained an appreciation of how your various systems function and how participation in regular exercise supports and improves the ways in which they operate. You now are familiar with ways in which the circulatory, respiratory, immune, muscular, skeletal, and nervous mechanisms serve you and how they and exercise are interdependent.

Second, after making your way through the book, I expect that you've come to understand what the term exercise really means, and moreover, why it not only has to be done regularly but also *sensibly*. I have emphasized this word, *sensibly*, repeatedly with hope that when planning a program of physical activity you would do so insightfully and in accordance with the many cautions and guidelines I've provided.

During your reading you've undoubtedly encountered new and perhaps even provocative ideas, but perhaps after some reflection you've decided to integrate them comfortably into your approach to living. Perhaps you've even begun to do so. A case in point would be the notion of *wellness* and the ways in which it differs from the old standby, *health*. This distinction aside, I trust you now appreciate the ways in which regular participation in exercise benefits both conditions. Yet another critical term that was explained in detail is *fitness*, clearly one of the book's foundational concepts. And of course, all of my discussions and treatments have been offered with an eye toward aging.

I've encouraged you to be conversant with a number of human experiences described in the book so your lives can be enriched and lived fully and enjoyably. I've introduced the notions of *stress* and *anxiety*, and shown how they differ and how they may be profitably managed through exercise. I've talked about the energy underlying all of our behaviors, the veritable charge that impels behavior in any particular direction, namely *motivation*. I have dwelled upon the importance of this powerful force that's necessary not only to embark upon, but also maintain regular adherence to your physical activity regimen. Chapter 4 was devoted to clarifying psychological factors that either underpin or interplay with exercise. Various terms and theoretical approaches to understanding motivation were reviewed in an effort to clarify stick-to-it-iveness.

In Chapter 3 you were introduced to the connections between what you eat and your wellness, health, and fitness. We talked about fat and fatness and its relationship to exercise, understanding full well that a common motivation for physical activity is bodyweight regulation. Chapter 5 was devoted to injury. Cautionary procedures and potential and avoidable errors in planning and executing exercise were reviewed.

Lastly, in Chapter 9, specific guidelines were provided that should be valuable in constructing your very own exercise program. And for those of you who think you might enjoy competition or organized programs of exercise involving other participants, I've included a number of suggestions, alternatives, and opportunities.

I wish you good fortune, good luck, good health, high wellness, and profitable and enjoyable exercise.

Do it. Move it—now!

GLOSSARY

A

aerobic—occurring in the presence of oxygen, aerobic activities proceed with the intake of environmental air (which contains oxygen)

aerobic exercise—physical activity done with the ready availability of an oxygen supply (walking while inspiring environmental air is an example)

Alzheimer's disease—form of dementia caused by plaque interspersed among nerve cells in the brain

anorexia nervosa—eating disorder involving voluntary near-starvation, often accompanied by highly excessive exercising

antigravity muscles—that part of the muscular system responsible for ensuring the upright posture, muscles that attempt to countermand the effects of gravity

alveoli—tiny air sacs that compose the lungs

appetite—psychologically based desire to seek and eat food

arterioles—very small arteries involved in transporting blood to the body's various organs and tissues

arteriosclerosis—condition affecting arteries, resulting in their hardening and loss of flexibility

arthritis—disease of the joints that comes in two kinds: rheumatoid and osteoarthritis

axon—long part of the nerve cell that carries messages from the cell body to the dendrites (nerve endings)

B

beta-endorphin—neurotransmitter (biochemical) produced in the brain and found in the blood stream, which has its concentration increased by exercise and is responsible for a feel-good response

biceps muscle—skeletal muscle that when contracted flexes the arm (lower arm brought toward upper arm)

biochemicals—chemical substances found throughout the body and generated by body tissues

blood vessel—tube-like structure of varying diameters and lengths that carries blood to or from the heart

body image—evaluative self-view of the body, way in which one views his or her physical self

body mass index (BMI)—formulaic method of determining the amount of stored body fat

bulimia—eating disorder involving gorging of food followed by purging

C

capillaries—minute, thin-walled blood vessels scattered throughout the body

carbon dioxide—waste gas, product of cellular metabolism

cardiorespiratory—interaction of two physiological systems: the cardiovascular (heart and blood vessels) and the respiratory system

cholesterol—A waxy substance found in the blood or in the walls of blood vessels, about 20% of which is contingent upon dietary intake

circadian rhythms—physiological variations within an individual occurring throughout a 24-hour cycle

circulatory system—composed of heart, arteries, and veins operating in conjunction with one another to distribute blood throughout the body

cognition—mental activities such as thinking, remembering, learning, and utilizing language

collagen—type of tissue responsible for plumping up the skin, which tends to decrease in volume with age

connective tissue—soft (nonskeletal) tissue that supports or connects bones, ligaments, and tendons

coronary heart disease (CHD)—conditions afflicting the heart such as heart attack, stroke, and arteriosclerosis

cortisol—product of the cortex of the adrenal gland which increases in concentration stressful (emotional or physical) experiences

CT scan—diagnostic procedure that combines individual X-ray images into a unitary three dimensional picture (computed tomography)

D

dendrite—small, thin, hair-like terminal processes of the nerve cell into which the axon transmits its neural message and which, in turn, relays the received message to dendrites of adjacent nerve cells

dementia—condition in which cognitive processes are significantly compromised

diabetes mellitus—disease involving inadequate secretion or utilization of insulin, excessive amounts of sugar in the blood, excessive amount of urine production

DNA (deoxynucleic acid)—building blocks of genes

digestive system—one of eight bodily systems that has as its primary function to break down ingested foodstuffs and distribute their nutrients to the body's cells

distress—stress reaction unfavorable to the individual

dopamine—neurotransmitter (biochemical) produced in the brain and found in the bloodstream that renders a feel-good response and increases in concentration with exercise *dynamic stretching*—stretching that mimics movement of the body (contraction or extension of the muscles involved in a particular physical activity), elongation of skeletal muscle in preparation of motor activity

E

endocrine system—one of eight bodily systems, which tissues are responsible for manufacturing and distributing essential hormones that regulate various metabolic processes

enkephalin—neurotransmitter (biochemical) produced in the brain and found in the bloodstream that increasees in concentration with exercise and is responsible for the feel-good response

ergogenic—stimulus that inspires work or effort

environmental stimuli—perceived changes in the external environment

enzymes—chemicals produced in special body cells and necessary for the regulation of various metabolic processes

essential vitamin—a vitamin that is necessary to the diet in order to avoid disease

eustress—stress reaction that is favorable to the individual

excretory system—one of eight bodily systems, which has as its primary responsibility the discharge of waste materials from the body

expiration—process by which waste gas is excreted from the body and shunted into the external environment (breathing out)

extrinsic motivation—motivation originating from sources external to the individual

F

fast-twitch muscle cell—muscle cells that contract rapidly during sustained physical activity *fatigue*—condition of weariness as a result of physical exertion

fiber—form of carbohydrate not broken down by the body's natural chemicals, it passes through both large and small intestines undigested

fitness—condition in which the physiological and neuro-muscular requirements of typical daily needs are satisfied

G

genetic makeup—idiosyncratic genetic profile within each person that determines his or her innumerable structural and functional characteristics

glucose—blood sugar required for proper functioning of body cells

H

health—degree to which all bodily systems and mental states are illness-free, sound, and functioning properly.

hormone—any of a number of chemicals produced by the endocrine system and shunted via tubules directly into the blood stream

hunger—physiological-driven desire to eat, typically occurring when the stomach is empty

hypertension—high blood pressure

I

immune system—one of eight bodily systems with the purpose to defend against foreign substances that may invade the body and possibly do it harm

inhalation—process by which environmental air is brought into the body (breathing in)

intrinsic motivation—motivation originating within an individual's psychological framework

introversion—behavioral tendency to be inwardly directed

J

jogging—slow running, usually considered to be at a pace no faster than eight minutes per mile

joint—anatomical junction where two or more parts of the skeletal system (bones) interact

L

ligament—tissue that connects a bone to another bone

long-term memory—memory holding information relating to events that occurred in the distant past

M

magnetic resonance imagery (MRI)—diagnostic procedure utilizing various radiation frequencies designed to reveal diseased body tissues

major minerals—phosphorous, calcium, magnesium

max VO₂—volume of environmental air able to be introduced to the body and processed by the lungs and respiratory system

melanin—fatty coating covering and thus insulating the axon of the nerve cell

METs (metabolic equivalents)—units of measurement used to express the maximum degree of exercise a person can accomplish

metabolism—sum of all processes by which cellular energy is produced; the sum of cellular processes that involves changes in the body's cells (building up and tearing down of the cellular material)

mind—thinking or cognitive function of the nervous system

modeling—process that influences observable behavior, emotional responses, and cognition that involves utilization (copying) behaviors executed by another or others; replication of what another person does *moderate physical activity*—exercise that burns 3.5–7.0 kilocalories per minute and results in 60–73% of peak heart rate

moral victory—competitive outcome perceived by a participant or participants to be somehow favorable despite a loss

motivation—force or forces that energize a particular behavior or set of behaviors, factors that account for behavioral directions or strengths

motor portion of the nervous system—that part of the nervous system responsible for carrying movement messages from the brain to the body's musculoskeletal system

motor stimuli—messages from the brain to skeletal muscles and connective tissue that initiate movement of the body

muscle rupture—tearing of muscle fascia (bundles) or muscle fibers

muscular contusions—muscle bruise usually due to physical trauma

muscular endurance—degree to which a muscle or muscle group is able to sustain a contraction (amount of time) or the frequency with which it is rhythmically able to repeat it

muscle strain—relatively minor tear or damage to a muscle or any of its fibers

musculature system—one of eight bodily systems, which comprises more than 300 muscles of various shapes, sizes, and functions

N

nervous system—one of eight systems that service the body, including the brain and myriad of nerves emanating from it that carry messages to all other organs and systems *neurogenerative disease*—disease involving some aspect(s) of the nervous system

norepinephron—chemical manufactured in the brain that stimulates the nervous system

neuromuscular—relating to the interaction of the nervous and muscular systems

neurotransmitter—chemical messengers that relay nervous impulses

O

optimal level of arousal—level of physiological activation that yields an optimal behavior, performance, or skill execution for a particular individual

organ—collection of like tissues that form a unitary structure dedicated to a specific bodily function (e.g., the liver, the heart)

osteoporosis—condition affecting the skeletal system that involves thinning or lessening of bone tissue

oxygen—gas brought into the body by the respiratory system, found in environmental air and essential to the basic metabolic processes

P

perceived exertion—degree of effort expended during exercise as interpreted by the exerciser

pectoral girdle—part of the skeletal system that supports the body's arms

pelvic girdle—part of the skeletal system that supports the body's legs

peristalsis—wavelike involuntary contraction of the smooth muscle lining the digestive tract that moves foodstuff onward

pernicious anemia—disease associated with the nervous system that involves the body's ability to absorb vitamin B-12

Pilates—prescribed series of exercises focused on the body's core (abdomen, lower and upper back, hips, buttocks, and thighs), devised by Joseph Pilates, that emphasizes stretching movements

plaque—fatty-like material that adheres to the inner lining of blood vessel walls

premature mortality—early death (earlier than actuarial data would predict)

pulse—rhythmic pounding of the blood against the walls of arteries that reflects the heart beat

R

reflex—automatic (no thinking or conscious decision making involved) response to an internal or external stimulus

respiration—combination of inhalation and exhalation processes

respiratory system—one of eight systems, comprises organs and tissues that form an organized mechanism for bringing in to the body environmental air, processing, and excreting waste gas

resistance training— physical activity regimen designed to increase muscular strength involving skeletal muscle flexion or extension against substantial weight (resistance)

running addiction—excessive and potentially harmful participation in physical exercise of some form and the emotional inability to disengage

S

self-concept—view held by an individual of all parts of the self

sensation-seeking—behavioral tendency to pursue situations and experiences that are physiologically activating

sensory portion of the nervous system—part of the nervous system responsible for carrying messages from the organs to the brain for processing *serotonin*—neurotransmitter (biochemical) produced in the brain and found in the bloodstream that renders a feel-good response, its concentration increased by exercise

short-term memory—working memory that holds information recently stored

slow-twitch muscle cell—muscle cells that contract slowly during sustained physical activity

skeletal system—one of eight systems, the bony framework that serves as levers for attached muscles, comprising more than 600 bones of various shapes and sizes

social psychology—subspecialty of the discipline of psychology, essentially concerned with interrelationships among people.

sun protection factor (SPF)—unit of measurement used to express the potency of sunscreen (protection against the sun's rays)

static stretching—stretching of skeletal muscle without moving body limbs, stretching that involves holding tension in the targeted muscle or muscle group for a predetermined period of time or until tension no longer exists

stress—unsettling reaction to events or factors occurring or having occurred in the internal or external environment

stress fracture—hairline break in bone tissue

subcutaneous fat—fat stored beneath the skin

synapse—junction of two or more dendrites where the transmission of messages occurs

system—collection of organs dedicated to a particular physiological requirement; for example, hundreds of bones of different shapes and sizes comprise the skeletal system

T

target heart rate—desirable heart rate during aerobic training *thermodynamics*—that part of the science of physics that deals with heat

thermodynamic theory of fat storage—scientific approach to understanding fat metabolism and storage based upon energy (heat/calorie) utilization

trace minerals—minerals that are needed by the body in small amounts

trachea—tube-like organ located at the rear of the throat and leading to the lungs

training—regular and systematic participation in exercise with the expressed purpose of improving physical fitness or some aspects of it

Transtheoretical Model—psychological framework for understanding the degree of an individual's readiness for embarking upon a beneficial regimen of exercise

V

visceral fat—stored fat located beneath the abdominal (underside) wall and surrounding some internal organs

veinule—very small vein involved in transporting blood back to the heart after it has serviced the body's organs and tissues

vigorous physical activity—physical activity that burns more than 7 kilocalories per minute and results in 74–88% of peak heart rate

voluntary muscles—muscles that are flexed or extended intentionally

W

weight training—system of training designed to develop or increase muscular strength that involves progressively increased resistance to targeted muscular contractions

wellness—state of being wherein all aspects of health are in balance; one can be well although afflicted with disease

REFERENCES

Alford, L. (2010). What men should know about the impact of physical activity on their health. *International Journal of Clinical Practice, 64*, 1731–1734.

Bailey, A. A., & Hurd, P. L. (2005). Finger length ratio (2D:4D) correlates with aggression in men but not in women. *Biological Psychology, 68*, 215–222.

Baker, L. D., Frank, L. L., Foster-Schubert, K., Green, P. S., et al. (2010). Effects of aerobic exercise on mild cognitive improvement. *Archives of Neurology, 67*, 13–14.

Berger, B. G., Pargman, D., & Weinberg, R. S. (2006). *Foundations of Exercise Psychology* (2nd ed.). Morgantown, WV: Fitness Information Technology.

Brody, J. E. (2008). Personal health. *The New York Times*, p. 7.

Brody, J. E. (2010). Personal health. *The New York Times*, p. 7.

Cohen, E. A., Ejsmond-Frey, R., Knight, N., & Dunbar, R. I. M. (2010). Rowers' high: Behavioral synchrony is correlated with elevated pain thresholds. *Biology Letters, 6*, 106–108.

Cohen, G. D. (2006). *The mature mind.* New York: Basic Books.

Dietrich, A., & Sparling, P. B. (2004). Endurance exercise selectively impairs prefrontal-dependent cognition. *Brain and Cognition, 55*, 516–524.

Emery, C., Kielcolt-Glaser, J., Glaser, R., Malarkey, W., & Frid, D. (2005). Exercise accelerates wound healing among healthy older adults: A preliminary investigation. *The Journals of Gerentology, 60*, 1432–1436.

Erikson, K. I., Prakash, R. S., Voss, M. W., Chaddock, L., Hu, L., Morris, K. S., White, S. M., Wojcicki, T. R., McAuley, E., Kramer, A. F. (2009). Aerobic fitness is associated with hippocampal volume in elderly humans. *Hippocampus, 19*, 1030–1039.

Ford, E. S., Bergman, M. M., Kroger, J., Schienkiewitz, A., Weikert, C., & Boing, H. (2009). Healthy living is the bet revenge: Findings from the European Prospective Investigation into Cancer and Nutrition—Potsdam Study. *Archives of Internal Medicine, 169*, 1355–1362.

Garland, T., Kelly, S. A., Malisch, J. L., Kolb, E. M., Hannon, R. M., Keeney, B. K., Van Cleave, S. L., & Middleton, K. M. (2010). How to run far: Multiple solutions and sex-specific responses to selective breeding for high voluntary activity levels. *Proceedings of the Royal Society B.*

Geda, Y., Roberts, R. D., Knopman, D. S., Christianson, T. J. H., et al. (2010). Physical exercise, aging and mild cognitive impairment: A population-based study. *Archives of Neurology, 67*, 80–86.

Greenberg, J. S., & Pargman, D. (1989). *Physical fitness: A wellness approach* (2nd ed.). Englewood Cliffs, NJ: Prentice-Hall.

Houston, A. I. (2010). Evolutionary models of metabolism, behavior and personality. *Philosophical Transactions of the Royal Society B27 Biological Sciences, 365*, 3969–3975.

Katz, J. (1993). *Swimming for total fitness—A progressive aerobic program*. Garden City, NY: Dolphin Books/ Doubleday & Co.

Kramer, A. F., & Erikson, K. I. (2007). Capitalizing on cortical plasticity: Influence of physical activity on cognition and brain function. *Trends in Cognitive Science, 11*, 342–348.

Lee, J., Dodd, M. J., Dibble, S. L., & Abrams, D. I. (2008). Nausea at the end of adjuvant cancer treatment in relation to exercise during treatment in patients with breast cancer. *Oncological Nursing Forum, 35*, 830–835.

Larson, E. B., Wang, L., Bowen, J. D., McCormick, W. C., Teri, L., Crane, P., & Kukull, W. (2000) Exercise is associated with reduced risk for incident dementia among persons 65 years of age and older. *Annals of Internal Medicine, 144*, 73–81.

Laurin, D., & Verreault, R. (2001). Physical activity and risk of cognitive impairment and dementia in elderly persons. *Archives of Neurology, 58*, 343–525.

Mahbuber, R., & Berenson, A. B. (2010). Accuracy of current body mass index obesity classification for white, black, and Hispanic reproductive-age women. *Obstetrics and Gynecology, 115*, 982–988.

Manning, J. T., & Taylor, R. P. (2001). Second to fourth digit ratio and male ability in sport: Implications for sexual selection in humans. *Evolution and Human Behavior, 22*, 61–69.

Nelson, M., Rejeski, J., Blair, S., Duncan, P., Judge, J., King, A., Naccera, C. A., & Castaneda-Sceppa, C. (2007). Physical activity and public health in older adults. Recommendation from the American College of Sports Medicine and the American Heart Association. *Circulation, 116*, 1094–1105.

O'Connor, J. (2010, September 1). Stefaan Engels runs a marathon a day, every day, 207 and counting. *National Post*. Retrieved from http://news.nationalpost.com/2010/0 9/01/stefaan-engels-runs-a-marathon-a-day-every-day-207-and-counting/

Pargman, D. (2007). Psychological bases of sport injury (3rd ed.). Morgantown, WV: Fitness Information Technology.

Pargman, D. (2006). *Managing performance stress: Models and methods*. New York, NY: Routledge.

Paul, S. N., Kato, B. S., Hunkin, J. L., Vivekanandan, S., & Spector, T. D. (2006). The big finger: The second to fourth digit ratio is a predictor of sporting ability in women. *British Journal of Sports Medicine, 40*, 981–983.

Prochaska, J. O., DiClementi, C. C., & Norcross, J. C. (1993). In search of how people change: Applications to addictive behaviors. *Journal of Addictions, 5*, 2–16.

Raglin, J., & Morgan, W. P. (1987). Influence on exercise and quiet rest on state anxiety and blood pressure. *Medicine and Science in Sports and Exercise, 19*, 456–463.

Ratey, J. (2009, October 8). Interview by Medscape. *Psychiatry and Mental Health*.

Ravaglia, G., Forte, P., Lucicesare, A., Piscane, N., Rietti, E., Bianchin, M.,

& Dalmonte, E. (2008). Physical activity and dementia risk in the elderly. Findings from a prospective Italian study. *Neurology, Part 2, 70*, 1786–1794.

Romero-Corral, A., Sommers, V. K., Sierra-Johnson, J., Thomas, R. J., Collazo-Clavel, M. L., Korinek, J., Allison, T. G., Batsis, J. A., Sert-Kuniyoshi, F. H., & Lopez-Jimenez, J. (2008). Accuracy of body mass index in diagnosing obesity in the adult general population. *International Journal of Obesity, 32*, 959–966.

Ryan, R. M., Weinstein, N., Bernstein, J., Brown, K. W., Mistretta, L., & Gagne, M. (2010). Vitalizing effects of being outdoors and in nature. *Journal of Environmental Psychology, 30*, 159–168.

Spirduso, W. W., Poon, L. W., & Chodzko-Zajko, W. (2008). *Exercise and its mediating effects on cognition*. Champaign, IL: Human Kinetics.

Spirduso, W. W., Francis, K. L., & MacRae, P. G. (2005). *Physical dimensions of aging* (2nd ed.). Champaign, IL: Human Kinetics.

Spielberger, C. D. (1972). *Anxiety: Current trends in theory and research*. New York: Academic Press.

Stark, S. D. (2000). *The stark reality of stretching* (4th ed.). Richmond, British Columbia: Stark Reality Publishing.

Wellness Letter (2010, July 26). University of California.

Trombetti, A., Hars, M., Hermann, F. R., Kressig, R. W., Ferrari, S., & Rizolli, R. (2010). Effect of music-based multitask training on gait, balance, and fall risk in elderly people. *Archives of Internal Medicine, 170*, 1794–1803.

Werner, C., Furster, T., Widman, J., Poss, J., Roggia, C., Hanoun, M., Scharhag, J., Buchner, N., Meyer, T., Kindermann, W., Haendler, J., Bohm, M., & Laufs, U. (2009). Physical exercise prevents cellular senescence in circulating leucocytes and in the vessel wall. *Circulation, 120*, 2438–2447.

Williamson, J., & Pahor, M. (2010). Evidence regarding the benefits of physical exercise. *Archives of Internal Medicine, 170*, 124–125.

Wolin, K., Yan, Y., Colditz, G. A., & Lee, I. M. (2009). Physical activity and colon cancer prevention: A meta analysis. *British Journal of Cancer, 100*, 611–616.

INDEX

A

aerobic capacity, 9–10
aerobic exercise, 192–193
aging
    attitude toward, 80–81
    and the brain, 83
    as a continuum, 89–90
    and labels, 88–89
    and memory, 95–96
    and nervous system changes, 93–94
    and psychological changes, 92–93
    and reaction time changes, 94–95
American Senior Fitness Association,
    205–206
anxiety vs. stress, 131–132
appetite vs. hunger, 66
aquatic exercise, 201–202
arousal
    and performance, 133–134
    and stress, 132–133
arteriosclerosis, 72
arthritis, 17

B

balance, 32–34
behavioral changes. *See* Transtheoretical Model
biceps muscle, 18
body image, 57–59, 85–86, 159–160, 171
bone density, 33
BMI (body mass index), 67–68
brain vs. mind, 86–87

C

caloric requirements, 67
cancer
    of the colon, 49–50
    prevention of, 50
    studies involving, 30–31
carbohydrates, 71
cholesterol, 72, 76
circuit training, 195–196
circulatory system, 7–12
collagen, 29–30
competitiveness, 141–143
cortisol, 27–28
cross training, 198–199
cycling, 196

D

dementia, 3
diabetes, 51–52
digestive system, 66

E

eating disorders
    anorexia, 64–65
    bulimia, 65
endurance exercise. *See* resistance training
evaluating individual needs, 182–184
exercise
    addiction to, 139
    aerobic vs. anaerobic, 13
    and the brain, 3, 83–84
    clothing for, 157–159, 160, 197
    definition of, 6

and memory, 96–97
and mood change, 83–85
physical benefits of, 34
and respiration, 19–20
scheduling of, 173–174
social benefits of, 97–100, 119–120
exercise machines, 194

F

falling, 31–32, 34
fat
    in culture, 61
    and exercise, 23–25
    as a nutrient, 72
    storage of, 59–60, 61–64
fatigue, 20
fiber, 71
fitness
    definition of, 6
    goals, 42–44
    and memory, 87

G

glucose, 51
goal setting, 167–169
goal-setting steps, 169–177

H

HDL. *See* high density lipoprotein
heart rate. *See* pulse
high density lipoprotein, 11
hormones, 27–28, 51
hunger vs. appetite, 66
hypertension, 4, 23–24

I

identifying physical capabilities, 91–92
illness, 38–39
immune system, 25–28
injury
    avoidance of, 109–111
    definition of, 104
    due to environmental factors,
        108–109
    due to improper movement, 105
    due to inappropriate exercise, 105
    due to psychological factors, 106
    due to subconscious factors, 107

recuperating from, 116–119
    types of, 111–113, 115–116
insulin, 51

J

jogging, 196, 197–198, 199–201

M

max VO2, 13–14
memory
    and aging, 95–96
    and exercise, 96–97
    and fitness, 87
    types of, 95–96
metabolic equivalents, 11
metabolism, 13, 20
METs. *See* metabolic equivalents
minerals, 75–76
modeling exercise behaviors, 162–163
motivation
    achievement and sustainment of,
        154–157
    definition of, 152
    and music, 161–162
movement patterns, 4
muscles involved in activities,
    184–185, 186–187
muscular system, 18–19

N

National Senior Games, 205
nervous system, 14–16
nutrition vs. diet, 57

O

osteoporosis
    definition and symptoms of, 48
    prevention of, 49
oxygen, 12–13

P

perceived exertion, 10
pilates and yoga, 114, 189–190
plaque (arterial), 7–8, 11, 72
protein, 72–73
pulse, 9

R

realism in creating exercise programs, 187

relationships between body systems, 16

resistance training, 190–192

respiratory system, 12–14

road races, 200–201

running, 196, 197–198, 199–201

running addiction, 45

S

self-concept, 58–59

senior centers, 206

senior exercise programs, 203–206

Senior Games, 204

Silver Sneakers, 204

skeletal muscles, 18

skeletal system, 16–17

skin, 28–31

sport as exercise, 139–140

stages of development, 90–91

strength exercise. *See* resistance training

stress

and arousal, 132–133

definition of, 125

learning-orientation approach to, 128–129

management of, 135–136, 137–138, 144

personality approach to, 129–130

psychodynamic approach to, 127–128

social/environmental approach to, 130–131

types of, 126–127

vs. anxiety, 131–132

stressors, 125–126

stretching, 113–115, 187, 189

swimming, 30

T

target heart rate, 10

thermodynamic theory of fat storage, 63

Transtheoretical Model, 151–152

V

vitamins, 73–75

W

walking, 196, 197–198, 199–201

water, 69–71

wellness

components of (*see* wheel of life)

definition of, 39

wheel of life

imbalance in, 41–42, 43–44

segments of, 40–41

visualization of, 39–40

Y

YMCA, 205

yoga and pilates, 114, 189–190

ABOUT THE AUTHOR

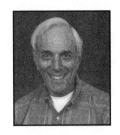

Dr. David Pargman is emeritus professor of educational psychology at Florida State University, where he served as program leader for educational psychology and coordinator for graduate studies in sport and exercise psychology. Prior to his 31 years of service at Florida State University, he taught at Boston University and the City College of New York. Pargman received a master's degree from Teachers College, Columbia University, and a PhD from New York University.

Pargman is author or co-author of six other books that deal with stress and performance, fitness and wellness, and sport psychology. He has been major professor to more than 40 PhD graduates and prior to his retirement was a fellow of the American College of Sports Medicine, the Association for the Advancement of Applied Sport Psychology, and the Research Consortium of the American Alliance of Health, Physical Education, Recreation and Dance. He is also a Certified Sport Psychology Consultant for the Association for the Advancement of Applied Sport Psychology and was listed in the United States Olympic Committee Sport Psychology Registry.

Pargman has served as visiting professor at the University of Akron, Ohio, USA; Srinakharinwirot University, Bangkok, Thailand; University of San Marcos, Lima, Peru; University of the Andes, Merida, Venezuela; Lund University, Lund, Sweden; and the University of Zulia, Maricaibo, Venezuela. He is currently on the Editorial Board of the Journal of Studia Kinanthropologia (Czech Republic) and the Board of Directors of the Multidisciplinary Institute of Neuropsychological Development (Cambridge, Massachusetts, USA).

Pargman was a member of his college track and cross-country team and has since competed in hundreds of road races.